A Better Second Half

Also by Liz Earle

A Better Second Half

Dial back your age to live
a longer, healthier, happier life

*Sharing my secrets to looking
and feeling better than ever*

Liz Earle

First published in Great Britain in 2024 by Yellow Kite
An imprint of Hodder & Stoughton
An Hachette UK company

1

Copyright © Liz Earle 2024

The right of Liz Earle to be identified as the Author of the Work has been asserted
by her in accordance with the Copyright, Designs and Patents Act 1988.

A CIP catalogue record for this title is available from the British Library

Hardback ISBN 978 1 399 72367 1
Audiobook ISBN 978 1 399 72369 5
ebook ISBN 978 1 399 72368 8

Typeset in Celeste by Hewer Text UK Ltd, Edinburgh
Printed and bound in Great Britain by Clays Ltd, Elcograf S.p.A.

Hodder & Stoughton policy is to use papers that are natural, renewable
and recyclable products and made from wood grown in sustainable
forests. The logging and manufacturing processes are expected to conform
to the environmental regulations of the country of origin.

Hodder & Stoughton Ltd
Carmelite House
50 Victoria Embankment
London EC4Y 0DZ

www.yellowkitebooks.co.uk

'Light tomorrow with today'
Elizabeth Barrett Browning
1806–1861

Contents

My Story

Some of you may have followed my more public journey over the decades, through pregnancies, brand-building, family health issues, divorce, hormone health and more. Others may be connecting with me here for the first time, so I'll give you a bit of background for context.

To begin at the beginning, I started work as a junior beauty writer in 1983 at a time when the world of wellbeing was really only just starting to open up. One of my early inspirations was the late, great Leslie Kenton, the groundbreaking health and beauty editor on the magazine Harpers & Queen (now called Harper's Bazaar). I remember seeing her at many press events and being in awe of this extraordinarily dynamic middle-aged woman, dressed in flowing white clothing, who exuded an esoteric glow as she extolled the benefits of juicing, raw foods and newly reawakened complementary therapies such as crystal vibrations, magnetic energy waters and reiki – the original Goop goddess. She was a visionary, a fearless pioneer, undaunted by being thought of as a bit of a quack and she heralded a new era of wellness journalism. Later, one of the highlights of my TV career was when she appeared as a guest on my own TV show, Liz Earle's Lifestyle, in the nineties. Back at the start of my career, *doyennes such as Leslie and other editorial gurus were generous in their sharing of knowledge and skills with a lowly junior writer, like me. There were many press trips that took me to far-flung places – argan oil extraction in Morocco, Hollywood beauty secrets in Los Angeles, longevity studies at Harvard Medical School, rose oil harvests in Turkey, the Oriental spas of Bangkok and beyond, as well as behind the scenes in Swiss research labs, French perfumeries, Eastern European thermal therapies and more. It was from those early assignments for both ITV and the BBC that I found my true passion for discovering ways to live well.*

In the early eighties, there was a small but growing band of seemingly weird and wonderful practitioners popping up on the UK alternative health scene – naturopaths, functional medicine specialists, nutritionists, acupuncturists, aromatherapists, detox advocates, juicers, qigong masters, herbalists, sound healers, energy workers . . . many of whom had obviously been around forever, but who began to gather more mainstream interest as 'alternative' or 'complementary' therapies became more talked about. It felt exciting and dynamic to be at the start of this New Age revolution in healthcare, a time when we, the public, were empowered to take a closer look at how the way we live affects our health and wellness.

I wasn't easily convinced at the beginning though. The first time I interviewed a naturopath who told me that my chronic eczema could be cured by changing my diet, I thought she was mad. Surely my skin would only respond to topical applications of ointments and unguents (in my case, years of prescription steroids). How could what I ate possibly have an external impact on my skin? Such was the perceived wisdom at the time – that conventional medication was the only way to fix dis-ease. Doctors were told to treat symptoms, not discover the cause (unfortunately, still often true today). In my case, the naturopath advised me to increase certain fats in my diet, cut out gluten, dairy and tomatoes (at least for a while), take evening primrose oil and specific vitamin supplements and drink a whole lot more water. Sceptical, I did as I was told and lo – my skin cleared, and has remained clear to this day (even though I do now occasionally eat some gluten and a lot of dairy, which happens to suit me).

My own experience of how we have the power to make such a dramatic difference to how we look and feel was a light bulb moment. The light flicked on. The penny dropped. We can indeed improve our bodies, brains (and beauty) by changing what we eat – and how we live. For me, the starting point was fats and oils. Back in the early eighties, TV diet gurus were urging us to strip all fats and oils out of our diets. These dietary macros were viewed as the very devil when it came to healthcare, intrinsically linked to weight gain and serious illnesses such as coronary heart disease (CHD) and stroke. Or so we were told. But my own experience told me otherwise. When I started to eat the right kinds of fats and oils (extra-virgin olive oil, essential fatty acids such as the gamma-linolenic acid (GLA) from evening primrose oil, real butter instead of hydrogenated synthetic margarine and other trans fats) not only did my eczema clear and my skin glow, but I also lost weight and felt more energised in the process. This led me to write my first book, Vital Oils, *which was counter-culture at the time, as mainstream medics and professional dieticians were urging low-fat eating (alas, many still do). I'll come back to this later, when I discuss diets and the foods we should be focusing on in more detail.*

Instead of following the popular narrative, I wrote about the dangers of low-fat as being damaging to our brains and bodies. I urged a switch back to real, whole foods such as grass-fed meat, sustainable fish and organic dairy. Loving the research, I moved from penning short-form magazine articles to writing books, where I discovered a genuine passion for unravelling complex academic research, distilling it into a more accessible form so that I can also better understand before communicating it to others. I've had some inspirational teachers and love few things more than connecting with great medical minds, often hidden away in the halls of academia and research labs, where so many mind-blowing health and wellbeing discoveries are made, not necessarily the media medics with their colourful Instagram accounts, PR agents and chat show circuits (although I do respect a select few). I'm referring to those clinicians and researchers quietly working away at the cutting edge of their specialisations, not out to sell us anything or launch some new product range – these are the unsung heroes of wellness. Their work often leads to some of the greatest discoveries, free from corporate agendas and commercial funding that can colour how information is presented. The internet can be a powerful and positive resource, but it's important not to rely on the University of Google and search-engineered 'science', finding instead independent voices, free from vested interests, whom we can trust. Hopefully, I can be one of these for you.

Writing about skin, researching natural ingredients, plant-based remedies and the like led me to co-found the Liz Earle Beauty Co., with my great friend Kim Buckland. Started as a sideline (it was actually Kim's idea, based on her industry experience), it quickly took off and I spent increasing amounts of time travelling the world, selling skincare. It was an exciting time to be brand-building and Kim and I built our business from a team of two across a kitchen table into a multinational, global brand – one of the largest independent beauty companies in the UK, in fact. But I was being pulled further and further away from my passion and purpose – writing and researching ways to live well. It reached a point when Kim and I (along with several other stakeholders) decided to sell the beauty brand, back in 2010, a date that worked especially well for me as it coincided with the birth of my last child. Once free from the constraints of the beauty company that still carries my name, I was keen to return to my first and foremost passion, so proceeded to write Skin, *a six-week inside-out plan for radiant skin;* The Good Gut Guide, *one of the first consumer books on the microbiome; and* The Good Menopause Guide, *also one of the very first books of its kind. I also launched my website, several social media channels,* The Liz Earle Wellbeing Show *podcast and bi-monthly magazine,* Liz Earle Wellbeing.

It was this immersion back into the world of wellness, many decades after the start of my career there, that got me back in shape both physically and mentally. Through writing and researching for my platforms, I realised how far I had fallen in terms of my own personal wellness. I learnt about the gut–brain axis, the effects of perimenopause, nutrigenomics, high-intensity weight training, low-carb diets, nootropics, cryotherapy, bio-hacking and more. I began to apply what I was learning to myself, using my own mind and body as a testing lab and sharing my results online. My shape changed. I lost weight, toned up, became physically stronger, emotionally more resilient, mentally happier and more purposeful. My skin changed, becoming plumper, more toned and less saggy than before. My hair grew back thicker and fuller, I had to start cutting my nails with scissors and they no longer flaked or developed the ridges of ageing. My cellulite pretty much disappeared and my sleep dramatically improved. I began to feel as though I was finally pulling myself out of a dulled state of disarray, up and out into the light; back into a world of optimism and hope, where I felt so much better able to cope with the challenges and the tough times all of us face all around us.

As I celebrated my sixtieth birthday in 2023, I became even more aware of the passing of time and its impact on my physique and psyche. I asked myself two fundamental questions:

1. *What do I need to do for myself now to live and age well?*
2. *How best to share what works to help others do the same?*

This book is the answer to those two simple questions.

I want to dispel the notion that we're all washed-up by midlife and that it's downhill after we hit 40, 50, 60 – or way beyond. There are so many positives to celebrate by the time we reach midlife – a gift denied to many. We know our own minds and we've accumulated many decades of wisdom and valuable life experience.

I genuinely believe that what is yet to come can and should be better than before, but we have to break the current narrative in order to let that happen. The process of ageing does not have to be downhill. I was stronger, fitter and more capable in my fifties than I was in my forties, so why can't I be even more so in my sixties, seventies and beyond? Who's to say we can't, or shouldn't, change the way we age? My wellbeing community consists of many thousands of midlife women (and many millions more through my social media, magazine and podcasts) and we share countless conversations on growing older. A common thread among those of us considered 'more mature' by society (frankly, a euphemism for being past it) is of losing our identities, of becoming invisible, feeling useless and worthless, a sense of redundancy – no longer needed by growing children, perhaps overtaken on the career ladder or abandoned by spouses trading us in for younger models. It enrages me to see midlife women so often cast aside, considered unattractive, unworthy or unproductive as their conventional beauty fades and declining hormones mean they are no longer usefully procreative, but also disadvantaged by weakened brains, bodies and bones.

It's tragic that at a time when we've given so much of our lives to others and finally have more time for ourselves, our bodies decide to take a downward turn and start letting us down. But there are many things we can do about this, as you'll read. Of course, men have their own issues with ageing too, but nowhere near the extent and detriment of those faced by women. And this book is unapologetically written for the Sisterhood.

Liz x
London, 2024

Introduction

Does growing older scare the pants off you? Are you fearful of losing your mojo – not to mention your mind? Have the hormonal changes during perimenopause, menopause or post-menopause left you feeling flattened? Is the creep of midlife weight gain a concern, yet you feel confused by conflicting dietary advice? Are your stress scores high, your sleep quality low and anxiety scaling off the charts? Perhaps you're dissatisfied with the way you feel or despairing of who is looking back at you in the mirror. Well, this book brings you solutions and will encourage, empower and equip you to live more fearlessly.

My purpose in this book is to help us *all* find the energy, resilience, enthusiasm, physical fitness and emotional strength to thrive through our second half of life. I want all of us to be the very best versions of ourselves, me included, no matter what our starting point is.

Much of what I'm sharing here has been learnt over 35 years of researching and writing within the world of wellbeing.

I've been fortunate to connect with literally hundreds of experts over the years, genuine specialists in their own areas of expertise and knowledge. I've done all the research into how to have a better second half so you don't have to and, throughout this book, I'll be offering the headlines and highlights on everything from hormone health and menopause matters to brain health, physical fitness, ageing, dermatology, diet, nutrition, sleep, stress management, weight loss, relationships, functional medicine, bio-hacking and so much more.

I'm enormously grateful to have had access to such a dynamic database; a strong and super-informed wellness community which has shaped me.

Now it's time to give back and pass on much of what I've learnt, experienced and found to be true.

**Take care of your body and your self –
it is the only place you have to live.**

This is the book I want *all* women to read. It's my midlife manifesto. I want my daughters to read it – and your daughters, and your friends and the women you work with. In fact, any woman who matters to you needs to read this book.

Life is difficult; that much we know. And midlife women are often hit the hardest of all. Trust me, I've been there and it's not been easy to find ways through the fog and into the light. I don't mind admitting that I've come to realise much of what makes a difference relatively late in life (better late than never). I struggled through my forties with fluctuating hormones during perimenopause; felt the toll on my body of having my last of five children late in life, aged 47; battled through the stress of selling a global beauty business – not to mention the loss of confidence and car crash of emotional wreckage when my second marriage broke down over many years before finally ending. Coming through all this and more besides, I can hand-on-heart say that, today, I have never felt happier, fitter, stronger, wiser, more joyful and positive about myself and the future than I do right now. And I want to share this wonderful place. A place where we're more than content to be in the skin we're in. A place filled with glee at the glorious-ness of life and all it has to offer (OK, so I don't feel gleeful every moment of every day, but I do feel far better than I used to and there are definitely more than glimpses of glee most days now). The ongoing goal for myself, as well as for all of you reading this book, is to share safe, simple and effective ways to be better than before, to enjoy and embrace this mid-stage of life. Ultimately, to age well.

The Indian–American guru investor and philanthropist Naval Ravikant said, 'to write a great book you must first become the book'. **I am this book**. Everything I write here has helped shape me into who I am now, feeling fitter, happier and more 'sorted' with each passing year.

Regardless of your age or stage of life right now, whatever life has chucked your way, whatever disasters have befallen you or bad times you've had to put up with for too many years, you, too, can take back control, make a genuine difference to your health and wellbeing, and, above all, make life *so much better*. This book is about recon-necting with the stuff that actually matters – and is my tried-and-tested take on how to get the best out of this gift called life. Ultimately, it's about how to have a better second half; how to *thrive* and not just survive. I'll be covering much of the big stuff – physical health, emotional wellbeing and resilience – as well as some of the more superficial niceties, such as how we look. Call me shallow, but I do actually care about my skin, my hair, my nails. And, like for many, my weight and appearance have been a bit of a lifelong preoccupation, driven more by how I wanted to present myself to the world and not necessarily for reasons of better health. In some ways, the years of being highly visible on television, in magazines and on social media were an unhelpful motivator, making me place too much emphasis on how I look and not enough on how I feel. So along with finding the best ways to look good, I'll also spend some time exploring how to better support your midlife brain health and emotional wellbeing too. As is my passion, I'll be covering the day-to-day stuff that crucially supports these pillars, such as how to eat well, move well, sleep well and, ultimately, live well.

This book is also about future-proofing your wellbeing. It's about how you can live a better and, by default, more fulfilled, lighter (and, dare I say it, more playful) life. It isn't about living forever (although longevity definitely plays a part), it's about living your very 'best life', before the opportunity passes you by. It will equip you with the knowledge and tools you need right now.

I only wish I'd learnt a lot of this sooner. It would have saved me a great deal of personal angst, anxiety and heartache.

Now Is Our Time to Shine

Personally, I can't wait for the next stage of life. With more knowledge about myself, greater confidence in my abilities and more free time as my children fly the nest, I'm better able to nurture the things that matter to me personally and the close circle of friends I've grown to know, love and trust over the years. For those at a similar age and stage of life, this should be the moment when we feel our fittest and strongest (physically and emotionally), ready to reap the rewards of many years of putting others before ourselves, whether bringing up children, supporting spouses, caring for elderly relatives and/or investing enormous energies into our work lives and careers. Maybe you've done some or all of these and more. Well, now it's *your* time.

Perhaps secretly you feel it's too late, you've gone too far down the wrong path to make a difference or maybe you think the things I'm going to share with you won't work. Well, let me tell you straight: no matter who or where you are, or what stage of life you're at, you're plain wrong.

It's never too late to make a positive change for the better and to be the best version of yourself.

I don't say that lightly. Of course, I've made mistakes, as I'll share. I've messed up through a lack of awareness and taken a fair few unhelpful paths in life. Frankly, who hasn't? But I've also worked through these to get back on track, stronger and fitter than ever. Whatever you're going through right now, you can effect positive change. Don't lose sight of that.

Having the right mental attitude and approach to ageing is vital for success – believing you can take some control and make those first few steps towards a goal is the single most important part of your journey. I want you to truly believe that it's never too late, that you *can* and you *will* make a difference to how you look and feel in your later years. This positive mindset is going to be critical to your success and sustain you through the inevitable setbacks and potential pitfalls encountered along life's path. We all fall over or have bad days, but ageing well is too important to let this diminish your motivation.

Let's shed the things that we've been too scared to try or have held us back, and unlock the secrets to living life successfully, in the fullest sense. Not just financially or how we're judged by the world around us, but delve deeper into what *really* matters to us and discover how we can move on with the self-care, bodily respect and self-love we deserve.

A life in balance

My years working in wellbeing have taught me that it's about living life in a daily, achievable balance. The one thing that counts above all else? Consistency. It doesn't have to be much and it doesn't have to be hard, but it does have to be consistent.

Throughout this book I'll be encouraging you to adopt some simple health habits that become the norm for your life; a workable routine that fits into the way you live. The key is to get the *right* routine and then to stick with it. We all have bad days and fall off the wagon from time to time. I have many days when I make mistakes, do no exercise, lie-in late, miss deadlines, eat too much cake and drink too much tequila . . . but I tend to live by the 80:20 rule, doing the best I can 80 per cent of the time and allowing 20 per cent for cheats.

I hope you find the practical information in these pages helpful for your own life journey, as you navigate yourself into the future.

This is OUR TIME! Let's shine.

Ten Things I Wish I'd Known in My First Half

Before we begin, these are the ten things I wish I'd known to be true earlier on in my life. It's taken me some time to realise the enormous value of each one of these – and just how fundamental they are to live our best lives. Enjoy the shortcut.

1. Prioritise YOU

Attitude is ALL. Prioritise you for a change and start putting yourself first. It's like they say on the plane – put on your own mask before you help others so you're better able to assist them. Mindset matters from the outset. Set yourself up for success. You have to want to do this, for you. Take it one step at a time. Small wins add up to big gains. The better version of you that you become, the better able you are to make a difference to those around you. Self-care is not self-ish and healthcare matters as we age, especially when it comes to how well we physically and mentally age, improving our resilience, happiness and overall longevity.

2. Health and hormones cannot be ignored

Health is wealth and so much of our overall health comes from how we live. Our daily health habits make a difference. Genetics and family history play a part for sure, but the emerging science of epigenetics (how behaviour and environment can influence the expression of our genes) reveals we have much more authority over our genetic traits than we might assume. This is good news! Hormones are also the fundamental drivers of female wellness. They control our physical, mental and emotional health. Hormones heal us, in particular, oestrogen (often given the US spelling 'estrogen' online or in medical journals), alongside progesterone and testosterone – the three feminine fuels that help us age well.

3. What goes into our mouths makes a difference

What we eat (and drink) is the biggest health choice we have control over. Forget genes, personal circumstances and financial status, every day we alone decide what we're going to put into our systems for sustenance. I find that hugely empowering (given the right knowledge).

4. Gut health matters

The microbiome has been described as the most newly discovered organ in the body. We have millions more microbes than cells in our bodies and they affect every single aspect of us. They are the ultimate multitaskers, controlling just about everything you can think of – our brains, bones, skin, digestion, mood, sleep, weight loss, immune system, stress; you name it, the microbial to-do list is endless. Look after your gut bugs and they will look after you.

5. Brain health matters

The brain not only controls how we think, but also runs our physical selves too. We know the gut–brain axis governs mood and emotion, sleep, stress and immune response. Cognitive decline is terrifying. Rates of Alzheimer's disease and dementia (especially among women) are on the rise. But there are so many helpful ways we can bolster our brains with simple health hacks, newly discovered nootropics (also known as 'smart drugs' or cognitive enhancers), meditation and more.

6. Movement matters

Our bodies are designed to move, and getting older is no time to slump on the sofa with a pack of Pringles. Sitting is the new smoking – it's a killer. That's especially true for women. The only way to retain strong, well-toned muscles and bone strength is by exercise. It doesn't have to be for long, but it does have to be intense (like lifting weights or resistance exercise) and regular (two to three times a week, every week). For fitness, strength and shape, when it comes to our bodies, it's a case of use it or lose it.

7. Sleep is our silent superpower

We ignore getting good rest at our peril and prioritising sleep is top of my longevity wellness list. Getting a good sleep routine sorted is one of the fastest ways to transform our mental and physical wellbeing, from lowering stress and anxiety to speeding weight loss and supporting greater gut health. Rest is also rejuvenating and taking time for it needs to be a priority, not a pastime.

8. Relationships rule the world

This means our relationship with ourselves as well as those around us. Humans are social beings, designed to love and have family and friends. Broadening our social connections is crucial when it comes to ageing well. Now is the time to expand our horizons, by developing new skills and widening the circle of those we share them with. Now is not the time to shrink from our surroundings; it's a time for greater sociability and togetherness – and never forget that loneliness is a killer.

9. Consistent healthy habits are key

How to sum up good health in one word? Consistency. As I said, consistency is key, especially when it comes to the small stuff. Getting into good habits, from drinking more water, embracing the outdoors first thing in the morning, taking a cold shower and getting to bed earlier are all small steps, but added together they make a massive difference. Setting up a positive routine of non-negotiables has never been more important than in our second half of life.

10. A sense of purpose is what drives you

Why are we here? What's the point? Is the world a better place for us being in it? What will our legacy be and who would miss us if we were gone tomorrow? These questions are the daily drivers that determine our future happiness. Find your passion and your purpose before it's too late. End of.

CHAPTER 1

Prioritise You

Welcome to a new way of thinking about your health. If you follow my lead, you *will* discern a difference in the way you look and feel. You've already taken the most important and fundamental step, to be curious enough to examine what it takes to age well. Now my job is to persuade you that you actually want to do it. Deciding you're worth a little bit more time and effort is the first and most important part of the process. Even the longest and most challenging journey has to start with the first single footstep. So let's walk side by side, on a journey through the rest of our lives that is long, happy, fruitful and fulfilled.

Too many of us midlifers are plagued by weariness and fatigue, suffer unexplained symptoms, pop vast numbers of prescription pills or endure lengthy waiting lists for treatment. We're at an age when plenty can go wrong and lots will change in our bodies. It's easy to feel disheartened by it all. Perhaps things are not quite what you imagined they might be when you were in your 'invincible' twenties. Unforeseen life events, whether affecting us or those we're close to, will often bring us down. And once down, it can be hard to find the way back up again. We need to be mentally and physically robust enough to deal with the s**t that invariably hits us in some form – and not be defeated by it. It's not just ourselves either. Our children may have grown up and largely gone, but even as they leave us, they still return with their own problems that draw us in, inevitably affecting us too. We may be simply exhausted from caring for a spouse, partner, elderly parents or sick or dying relatives. This is part of the stage of life we'll often find ourselves at right now and it's understandable to feel overwhelmed by it all. Our best weapons of defence are physical strength and mental resilience. It's about being mentally and physically robust enough to deal with life's many challenges without either crumpling into a heap or internalising the stress, which can manifest later as our own chronic illness.

It's so easy to get to a stage where gaining good health can seem out of reach. Yet so much of what will make us feel better is actually very simple and well within our grasp for the taking. We can't control the things that happen to us, but we can control the way we respond to them. That alone is empowering. Better wellbeing is neither expensive nor complicated. In fact, the savings (and benefits) are huge when we know what to do, when and how. How best to start this journey through our second half? At the beginning.

Maybe the very thought of looking and feeling better than ever seems beyond you, and you feel almost defeated before you begin. If so, I'd like to offer some personal encouragement and share with you how my own health journey began.

I have not always looked and felt this well. By the time I reached my late forties I was seriously floundering in my work, my relationships and the way I looked and felt about myself. Physically, I was at my heaviest (nudging 12 stone) post-pregnancy and my least fit. I was struggling with work pressures and extreme overload, co-running the phenomenally successful Liz Earle Beauty

Company and witnessing my second marriage disintegrate along with the looks and vitality of my youth. I did not know it at the time, but I was in the midst of perimenopause, with crashing hormone levels causing anxiety, sleepless nights, lack of energy, low mood and weight gain. There's much talk about perimenopause and menopause now, which is such a good thing, but back then, it was all very hush-hush. Despite being a health and wellness writer for many decades, I hadn't even heard of the term perimenopause, let alone realised it was happening to me.

I'd been writing and researching health, beauty and wellbeing since my first job in magazine journalism in 1986, so you would have thought that I would have been better equipped and prepared for the great chasm of midlife angst that I found opening up in front of me. But it took a while for the penny to drop. I hope this book will help you to avoid this pit of despair and that I can fast-track you to a much better midlife – and far beyond. If you feel you're already descending downwards, allow me to pull you up and out.

Why Self-Care Matters

Life is precious. It is a priceless gift to be treasured. Our minds and bodies are things of wonderment. Our attitude to the way we take care of our most important personal assets is paramount. Do we actually appreciate what we have? Do we even bother enough about our brains and bodies to fuel them with nourishing food and drink? Or do we fill them with ultra-processed, commercial c**p because, deep down, we don't really care too much? Or perhaps we don't feel worthy of self-care? Well, forgive me for being blunt, but it's time we did care.

Let's be under no illusions here – midlife is hard. I know. During my middle years, I was someone else's wife, mother, daughter, sister, boss, colleague and friend. I gave my time to others but not to myself. Which in some ways is right and proper in a functioning society. Of course, we need to recognise our responsibilities and live up to them in the fullest way we can. But somehow along the way, our responsibility to ourselves can get overlooked. It's important to recognise the needs of others, but the many pulls on our time can become a bad habit, or at best a convenient excuse. We're just too busy looking after the kids, finishing that piece of work, spending time looking after other people ... often unwitting excuses for not getting out for some fresh air, not eating too well, short-changing our sleep or drinking more Chardonnay than we know we really should (guilty). If you feel a bit like this too, it's time to refund yourself some self-care. I'm not saying that it should suddenly be all about ME – but there's likely to be a need for a better balance, a recalibration of the way too many of us live our lives in order to thrive during, what should be, the very best years of our lives.

Today's generation are a lot savvier. I have two daughters, Brella in her early twenties and Lily in her early thirties, and they both talk about carving out 'me time' and the value of 'self-love'. But it's not too late for those of us who are older and more attuned to a different mindset.

Self-love is not self-ish.

I can say this now, but it's taken me years to appreciate the true value of my mind and body. I'm 60 years old (at the time of writing), have five fabulous children of whom I'm immensely proud and grateful for, successful businesses that bear my name and a thriving online community of incredible women curious for ways to live well, just like you. But until not that long ago, I was self-sabotaging my looks and energy levels by not taking enough personal care. Sure, I wanted to look and feel better, but I was suffering from that dreaded word – drift; just drifting along, making excuses as to why I didn't feel my best: I was stressed, tired, overworked, anxious, just didn't have the opportunity, the time, the resources ... But, ultimately, for things to shift and be successful you have to *really want it*. That means investing your time, your energy and your enthusiasm. Above all, it means commitment.

Do It for You

You are your number one priority. This is a bold statement, but we can't be either fulfilled for ourselves or most useful to others unless we've first looked after ourselves. This is wellbeing in the broadest sense. Be encouraged in this. The starting point has to be taking ownership of your health, even if you're battling something big.

Perhaps secretly you feel it's too late? Maybe your inner critic is telling you that you're just too far down the wrong path to be able to make a difference. Or maybe you think that the things I'm going to share with you are all well and good for *me*, but won't *really* work for you. Well, let me tell you straight – no matter who or where you are, or what stage of life you're at, it is **never** too late to make changes for the better.

There are always ways you can help equip your body for the very best chance for success, whatever that might look like for you.

As I said earlier, health is wealth and this is absolutely true – never more so realised than during the Covid-19 pandemic years, when our own mortality was put sharply into perspective on a global scale. Even the richest people on the planet have not been able to get around the fact that health is a non-negotiable asset. Regardless of our financial status or global superpowers, when it comes to priorities, how we care for the whole body – from brain to bones and beyond – is the most fundamental starting point.

I didn't start this journey until my mid-fifties. I wish I'd started sooner and I almost envy those of you in your thirties and forties who are picking up this book now. But it's not too late to make a difference at any age. How far you go with it is up to you. I'm not going to sit here and say that it's always going to be easy (although there are many helpful hacks and shortcuts), but believe me when I say it's worth it. Why? Because *you're* worth it (to borrow a line from another beauty giant)!

Reset Your Mindset

So much of who we are and what we do is governed by what's in our heads, not by our bodies. So this book is partly about unlocking and expanding your vision and daily mindset so you can be the absolute best version of yourself. For starters, stop comparing yourself to others. I've come to accept that there will always be someone cleverer, richer, prettier, younger (obviously!), slimmer, stronger, wittier, wiser and more capable than me. What matters is that I respect myself enough to be the best version of me. How? By taking the time and actually carving out some space in life to make this happen.

**It's time to be yourself –
everyone else is taken.**

Start by taking a moment to think about what's stopping you or holding you back. It's common to feel overwhelmed and powerless, but is that really the case? We can't always control what is happening, but we can control our response. That alone is empowering. Are we going to let a situation – or someone – define us? Or are we going to stop for a moment and consider our options? The starting point is to realise what is happening and to calmly consider what choices we have.

Take stock

Let's start by reassessing some priorities. The entry point for a better second half is to take stock of where we are here and now. What is your number-one priority right now? Is it you or are you somewhere at the back of the queue waiting for it to be your turn to be called? How do you feel about yourself and where you are in life? Are you happy and fulfilled, or feel that something is lacking? Do you look forward to older age with gleeful anticipation or a certain dread? Let's recognise and address regrets and failings, forgive ourselves for when we went wrong, let go of the grudges (real or perceived) and acknowledge what we could be doing better. The past is gone and largely irrelevant. It's time to live in this moment and to realise that NOW is the time to act.

Let's be honest with ourselves about what we'd like to be doing better, before even more time passes by. The longer we leave looking after ourselves, the harder it gets to make a meaningful impact. Start by making a list of the things you do well in life and those you could do better. Then take a hard look at those you feel you could improve – how many of these things really matter? If they're truly important, leave them on the list as room for improvement. If they're not fundamental to your future life, scrub them off and leave them for later (if ever). Of the things you do well, are they in the right order of priority? When I wrote my list, number one was work – my family came further down, followed by myself. It made me realise I was making the wrong decisions with my time – and I moved my family to the top. No one ever died wishing they'd spent more time on their emails.

Taking stock of life in our middle years is cathartic. As I get older, I think about how I could have reframed things in my life differently. I needed to rid myself of quite a lot of 'stuff' that wasn't doing me any good. I needed to exit a working environment that wasn't positive, leave a marriage that wasn't working and start to pay a lot more attention to getting both my physical and mental wellbeing in order. Looking back, it took me too many years to realise all of these things – precious time that was wasted for me, but perhaps helpful for you to think about now. Could I have spread the load a bit more, asked for help a bit more often, relied on others to help sort things out for *me* for a change?

Other people are not mind readers and often the simple act of telling someone what's troubling you will start the process of a better outcome. Don't be afraid to ask for help, be this from a family member, friend, colleague or even a healthcare practitioner. A problem shared is a problem halved.

It's time to take back some time for yourself and reclaim your personal power and autonomy. Share how you feel with those closest to you, start a journal if you feel hesitant – sharing thoughts and feelings with a pen and paper can be a useful first step. Get things off your chest and out of your head, even if that simply means writing them down where no one else will read them as a starting point. These are all things I wish I'd done sooner in life. I'm much better now at being more open about how I feel and reaching out for help, or asking friends if they'd mind if I simply had a rant and let off some steam. When all else fails, find a quiet space alone and have a good old shout at the universe – it's really very cathartic!

Before delving further into the pages of this book, take a moment to think about where to draw the line with what you're prepared to accept from those around you and what you yourself might need to receive from others. Do we have to do it all, all of the time? When is benign neglect of family members, household chores, the gardening acceptable, a good thing even? In the garden, I now accept that weeds are just plants growing in the 'wrong' place that can be left a while (wildflower meadows are essentially weed plots loved by pollinators), so my obsession with weeding is over. Can my older kids be left to sort out their own lunchboxes, shop for their own supper, do their own ironing (or wear crumpled clothes)? Yes? Excellent. My view is that if it's mostly OK, most of the time, then that's a good result. No blood and nothing broken? Good, so let's get on then.

How to Start the Day . . .

This chapter is entitled 'Prioritise You' and starting the day well has become my number-one wellbeing priority.

I've included this section here in detail because questions about my own personal routine are among the commonest I get asked:

Time for a reality check

Reading this, you're statistically likely to have family responsibilities and obligations, and our genetic female default is to care, nurture, aid and assist when we're asked to. But have we made this just a bit too easy for others? We've a tendency to 'helicopter', which is great for giving us a sense of self-worth but not so good for encouraging their independence. A better habit to adopt is to be open to anyone who has a problem to come to you, not only with the issue, but with at least a couple of ways in which they think it could be sorted out. Maybe we've got into the habit of being just that bit too available, of being the easy answer to those around us. Of course, being asked to sort something out also makes us feel needed and valued, so I do see that it's a fine line between being there for those who need us, whilst also encouraging a little more respect and self-sufficiency from those around us too. Just being a bit more aware of this can be very helpful.

'So what do you actually *do*?' 'How do you fit it all in?' 'What are the most important things I should be doing each day?' 'What supplements do you really take, how much, with what and when?'... the list goes on. I should start by saying that this is what I have found works for me, as your average, relatively healthy, middle-aged, Western-world woman. If this sounds more or less like you, then the chances are that this (or a slightly modified version of it) will work for you too. If not, there are still many helpful life lessons here, from dietary advice to guide us all, at whatever stage of life, to health hacks and habits we can *all* benefit from, whoever and wherever we are.

The first half an hour (and the last couple of hours) of the day are *the most important*. The first 30 to 60 minutes after waking is the time that sets us up for the day ahead. Depending on how we use this time, it will empower us to feel stronger, calmer and more capable of facing whatever life is waiting to throw at us. Even though I'm not naturally a morning person, I've come to realise that getting the day off to a good start is not just helpful, it's absolutely fundamental. If you are a morning person, lucky you – the morning really is the best time. Some talk about 'the power hour', but if I'm honest, I don't often have a full hour to spare (except perhaps on a Sunday morning or when on holiday) and I like my sleep far too much to get up before dawn, although that's something I'm working on . . . But I *can* grab 30 minutes, even on those days when the school run or an early train get me out of bed while it's still dark.

So this is my 30–60-minute morning routine that starts my day. Every day.

The first ten minutes
On waking, after a quick stretch in bed and a positive thought of gratitude (whatever I am facing that day, good or bad, I always thank God/the Universe for waking up safe and well), I head to the bathroom to weigh myself (without clothes). This is the lightest moment of the day – hurrah! Some people are against daily weighing, but I find it a helpful tool to keep track of where I am and how my body has responded to the day before. I'm not so bothered about how *much* I weigh (muscle weighs more than fat, so the fitter we become, the heavier we're likely to be), but I'm very interested in tracking change. Super-slim, super-fit athletes weigh much more than they're 'supposed'

to, according to body mass index (BMI) tables (a highly unreli-able measure – see page 169 for more on this), so we really shouldn't pay too much attention to these standard height/weight tables if we're getting stronger and converting fat to muscle. No, I'm more interested to see patterns of change and take early steps to shift a few excess pounds as they creep on, before they become permanent. The quicker we shift any extra pounds, the easier it is. That's why I weigh myself each and every morning. Some may find this obsessive; I find it works for me, but the choice is yours.

I'll then rinse out my mouth with water as my mouth can feel very dry on waking, dislodging the build-up of bad bacteria that cause our early-morning 'dragon breath'. I follow this with a quick bit of tongue scraping using a simple copper tongue scraper (find these online or in a health-food store). This is an ancient Ayurvedic technique of literally scraping away the layer of white fuzz that builds up on our tongues overnight. It's a very gentle and effective way to feel fresher and also provides an instant snapshot of our toxic load. I notice that when I fast (more on that later) my tongue is often covered with white fuzz as my body unloads its internal debris and waste cell matter (aka toxins). If you're run-down or have been drinking too much alcohol, you'll also notice this early warning sign on your tongue. It's a highly reliable indicator of what's going on, unseen, inside us. I follow tongue scraping with another good sloosh around with water and spit this out before brushing my teeth (once dead cell debris has been dislodged, it makes sense not to swallow it).

I follow this with a glass of water to refresh and rehydrate. Drinking plenty of hydrating fluids first thing should take priority before anything else. It's also a good way to get our water requirements in early on, in case we forget later on (which I tend to do, no matter how hard I try to remember). I drink filtered water, as filtering takes out much of the nitrates, chlorine and other chemicals that may be in the water supply, depending on your regional area.

To clean my teeth, I use a whitening formula toothpaste for sensitive teeth and an electric toothbrush, as this has been shown to help with gum health, which is especially important as we age and our gums recede. I also 'floss' with a Waterpik, or water flosser, most mornings, again to improve gum health. Regular flossing between the teeth helps remove harmful oral bacteria that have been linked with some serious diseases, including colon cancer and inflammatory bowel disease (IBD), where oral bacteria have been found deep in the depths of our intestines. This is due to the gum–gut axis transferring a build-up of bad bacteria in our gums to our digestive systems where they can cause harm. But it's important to go gently here, and using dental floss may not be as good for us as using a water flossing gadget, which delivers a pressured jet of water to clean between the teeth. Studies show a water flosser to be twice as effective as using dental floss, removing virtually all harmful dental plaque. Water flossers are also kinder on the gums and are unlikely to make them bleed, damage that creates a direct pathway for bad bacteria to enter the bloodstream. Water flossers also give a bit of gentle gum stimulation and I find them easier to access those hard-to-reach rear molars. Another good option is inter-dental sticks and here, I would choose the simple wooden variety over the un-eco plastic kind. Whichever form of cavity cleaning you choose, go gently and swoosh out your mouth with plenty of water afterwards so as not to swallow any of the bacterial build-up you've just dislodged.

The flaw of flossing

I definitely wouldn't use any kind of floss that has a non-stick 'glide' surface, coated in PFHxS chemicals (perfluorohexane sulfonic acid, to be precise), which have been linked with increased rates of heart disease and cancer. Harvard School of Public Health researchers found that women who flossed with these types of dental floss had higher levels of this chemical in their blood, probably due to the chemicals seeping into the gums (especially vulnerable when these bleed).

Never one to miss the chance to multitask, I practise improving my balance while brushing my teeth by standing alternately on one leg (30 seconds each side). Try this with your eyes shut to make it even harder! Balance is a really good indicator of how our bodies are ageing – the longer we can stand on one leg (preferably with our eyes shut), the younger our biological age. Or you may prefer to use this time to fit in a few squats or pelvic floor squeezes – anything that becomes a simple, healthy habit that makes good use of tedious toothbrushing time.

Rehydration

As I mentioned, first thing in the morning is the best time to rehydrate, and adding a glass of homemade electrolyte water (see page 190) gives the body an extra boost of energy. It's important to drink this *after* you've cleaned your teeth as it's quite acidic, especially if you make your own (as I often do) with fresh lemon or lime juice, which softens tooth enamel, so you don't want to be scrubbing your teeth just after drinking it. You can drink this through a straw if you prefer to protect your teeth or just rinse out your mouth with plain water afterwards. There's increasing talk in the wellness world about topping up our fluid intake with electrolyte drinks and it's something I've found to be a fast, cheap and easy way to give me a quick pick-me-up first thing, especially before exercise. It makes me feel instantly brighter and more alert. It's a simple early-morning health habit that works.

Journaling

I used to be a bit dismissive when it came to journaling. It's something my daughters are very keen on and I've interviewed a number of therapists over the years who are big fans, but somehow it never really resonated with me. I'm happy to report that I have changed my mind! I don't write lots of words, but do find that jotting down a few sentences and thoughts on how I feel first thing in the morning (and last thing at night) sets me up in a better way for the day ahead. I keep a pretty fabric-covered notebook beside my bed with a nice sharp pencil, and before my working day starts or I turn on my phone, this is what I write first thing:

- What I am grateful for and what would make the day look good for me.
- A few positive words of affirmation – the way I'm feeling about myself or how I'd like to be empowered to feel.
- A note of my weight and any other key metrics, such as pulse and blood pressure, I'm measuring out of interest. I especially do this when trialling new health hacks or ideas, to keep track of how my body is responding. I might add blood glucose levels or any other stats or vitals that some new app or gadget is suggesting I record.

I then leave space to make a note at the end of the day for the positive things that have happened, as well as anything that's circling around in my mind, troubling me like some bothersome fly, before bedtime.

These simple journal notes are a quick and easy health habit that take just a few moments but are surprisingly profound. I went away for a week's holiday and forgot my journal – and was struck by how much I missed it. Making notes on my phone was just *not* the same!

This is what my daily page looks like if you'd like to recreate your own notebook journal (or head to Useful Resources to find details of The Five Minute Journal):

Date ....

Morning

Vital stats ....

Today, I am especially grateful for ....

Affirmations: today I am ....

Evening

These good things happened today ....

These things are concerning me ....

Today I have learnt ....

The next ten minutes
Mind matters
Once I've put down my pencil and closed my notebook, I'll stretch out my back, arms and shoulders. Unless I'm in a tearing rush, I devote the next five to ten minutes to setting up my mind for the day ahead. Giving the brain a chance to cleanse itself is as important as taking a shower is for the rest of the body. It's such an important part of gathering in some calm mental clarity and resilience for the day ahead. For me, taking time out for a few minutes of meditation feels a bit like rinsing my brain under the tap. It's a vital bit of mental prep work for what lies ahead that day. And, as the saying goes, fail to prepare, prepare to fail.

I find a quiet space, such as sitting up on my bed or a corner of solitude downstairs, and use apps like Calm and Mindvalley, among others. It also helps to set your intentions at this time, to literally tell your mind what it's going to need to be doing for the rest of the day. Affirmations are helpful – phrases like 'I am strong, capable and calm' work well, or you may need some self-soothing, along the lines of 'I am OK, I can handle the difficulties I face, I am loved by God/the Universe/others', etc. You may have already written a few of these down in your journal. If you prefer, you can write them down again, or study the words in your notebook. Take a moment to focus on them, speaking these powerfully affirming words and phrases out loud or silently in your head. Either way, your mind will be listening.

I'm also newly into Vedic meditation, an offshoot of Transcendental Meditation, or TM (see page 236).

Do please try one of these meditative techniques before the day crowds in and you get distracted away from your innate, inner sense of peace. I find that if I don't do this simple routine first thing, I don't do it at all, which is a loss.

Supplementary benefits

Meditation done, I take my first supplements of the day. The first thing I take is a NMN, or nicotinamide mononucleotide, in the form of a white powder under the tongue. This gives energy levels a genuine boost (among other cellular protective and pro-ageing benefits). I feel a tangible lift after taking NMN and find it most useful to take early on. Some days I'll add in L-ornithine, an amino acid that helps reduce fatty deposits around the midriff (see page 182). This is a fussy supplement though and only works if taken on a *completely empty* stomach, so either needs to be taken last thing at night – a couple of hours after eating or drinking *anything* other than water or herbal tea (so no late-night glass of wine, nightcap or hot chocolate, for example) – or, for those who mostly eat late, like me, you can take it first thing in the morning, as long as it's before a brief bit of intense exercise (such as a minute or so of squats). The rest of my daily supplements I tend to take with food later in the day, to increase their absorption, and I'll list these when we look at diet in more detail (Chapter 4).

Get out, look up!

Those who follow me on Instagram will know that I also like to get outside really early on, either to sit outdoors for my above meditation (if the weather allows) or shortly afterwards and LOOK UP! I'll always face east towards the rising sun, to feel the fresh air and hopefully some sunshine on my face. I'll most often take a cup of black tea with me for company (I drink organic Earl Grey or a homemade chai brew – see my website for an easy recipe: lizearlewellbeing.com/healthy-food/healthy-recipes/drinks/home-made-masala-chai-tea). I look towards the sunrise as early as possible and am a believer in using the sun's energy to help set up our circadian rhythm for the day ahead (just as our ancestors did, long before the electric light bulb came along and changed our waking day forever).

Exposure to the sun's unfiltered rays first thing is increasingly recognised as an important part of our daily wellbeing. This is because the sun emits different forms of radiation throughout the day. This may sound counter-intuitive coming from someone better known for talking about protecting skin and warding off wrinkles as we age, but some sun exposure is positively beneficial. Bio-hackers talk a lot about the benefits of both early-morning and early-evening sunlight for getting our hormone balance straight. This is because the sun emits more blue light in the early hours and near infrared (NIR), which activates our pituitary gland and wakes us up (which is why we should avoid blue light emitting screens in the evening), and less of the skin-damaging ultraviolet radiation (the UVA and B rays that cause ageing and burning of the skin). Conversely, the sun emits more of the red light waves in the evening, which calm us down and encourage melatonin production before bed. Exposure to early-morning daylight (even when the sun isn't shining) improves our moods and emotional wellbeing as well as giving us a better night's sleep. Every cell in our bodies is influenced by the time of day as set by the sun, so not only are our circadian rhythms established for wake/sleep, but daylight also triggers hormone activity and has an effect on our trillions of gut microbes too, influencing everything from mental health to the immune system.

Interestingly, in-vitro (test tube) studies indicate that early-morning sun exposure may actually help better prepare the skin for the more damaging UV rays later in the day. This form of preconditioning the skin may even help protect it from burning later when exposed to stronger sunlight, with studies showing a reduction in erythema (redness) and post-inflammatory skin pigmentation. It's also been known for many years that low-energy exposure to these early visible and NIR wavelengths speeds cellular healing processes. This low-level light therapy has been used to hasten wound-healing and even reduce skin wrinkles, and has been compared to the form of plant photosynthesis which enhances energy production.

Personally, I feel my mood lift and am better set up for the day ahead if I can get outdoors early on and face the sun (even on a cloudy day), without using glasses, contact lenses – or sunscreen. Just don't leave it until the sun rises too high and never look directly into the sun as this will seriously damage the eyes. And when it comes to the skin, I always use mineral-based sunscreen on my face, neck and the backs of my hands when outdoors in the middle of the day or when the sun is strong (but I don't use it first thing).

Ten minutes on . . .

Get moving

Back indoors and it's time to work out and move my body. On those mornings when I have more time I may head to the 'gym', a converted garage at home, where I have a running machine, a bench and a few weights. Or I might do an online exercise class, a yoga session or head out for a short run. Even when time is tight, I will always (without fail and wherever I am) do a simple fitness regime, usually in my bedroom, often still in my pyjamas. This involves 100 deep squats, some hamstring and calf stretches, 60 fast push-ups (yes, these are a challenge but I tell myself it's just 60 seconds of your life, get over it), followed by 50 tricep dips and a few spine twists and shoulder rolls. No equipment required, so absolutely no excuses. See pages 245–49 for more detail on how and why to do these exercises. You'll find my simple early-morning routine on YouTube here if you fancy joining in: lizearlewellbeing. com/bshlinks

The benefits of 'grounding'

While getting outside to absorb those early-morning sunbeams, I also practise grounding. This is simply walking barefoot or lying skin-to-earth on the ground, preferably on grass. The premise is that the earth has an electromagnetic current that the body can tune into and benefit from. A convincing explanation is that connecting the body to the earth enables free electrons from its surface to transmit deep into the body, where they have an antioxidant and anti-inflammatory effect. If this all sounds a bit woo-woo, clinical studies show that grounding does improve wound-healing, possibly due to the earth's negative charge (ions) having a positive effect on cells around the damaged skin. These healing electrons may also more generally impact our immune systems and overall health. Grounding appears to improve sleep, regulate cortisol, reduce pain and reduce stress, as it shifts the autonomic nervous system (the fight-or-flight response) towards the parasympathetic (the quieter, rest-and-digest mode). Separated from the earth in everyday life by wearing synthetic-soled footwear, grounding may be one reason why we feel so much better on holiday, for example, when we're more likely to go barefoot. Give grounding a go – it is easy and free to do.

Shower time

Lastly, I jump in the shower, finishing with a minimum 60-second blast of icy cold water. This is a brilliant (free!) habit to get into for giving the body just the right amount of 'stress' to produce a useful cortisol spike. Yes, activating the hormone cortisol with a micro-stressor helps set us up for the day and supports the immune system, as long as it's first thing, not at night – and no more than a small stress spike.

And that's the first 30 minutes of the day done. No fancy equipment needed, no gym membership, totally portable, and can be done wherever you are, so again, no excuses.

If you've just read this and think 'no way do I have time for all this!' set your alarm for half an hour earlier and give it a go. Invest the first 30 minutes of each and every new day in YOU. What you set in place during the first half hour of every day has the power to carry you through the following 23.5 hours (and the rest of your life). Or not. The choice is yours. My advice is simple, if you do *nothing* else, prioritise this. Set yourself up for success. It works.

The Gender Divide

There's a growing awareness that many of our most common medicines such as painkillers (important, as more women than men take painkillers), statins (mostly tested on men), antibiotics and even cancer treatments may be inadequate for women because they've been primarily tested on men. This is especially true of some of the older drugs, such as paracetamol. Adverse reactions to drugs are the fourth biggest cause of death among older women, according to research presented to the EuroScience Open Forum back in 2010.

We know that women respond to medication differently because our stomachs may absorb medicines faster and our body fat distribution is different. Crucially, our female genes also play a significant role in how we respond to treatments, and new gender-specific cancer drugs are being developed to help address this disparity. This is an important point to make in the gender-changing debate, as we may decide to self-identify as a different gender, but we can't fundamentally change our chromosomes or alter the way some medications will affect our cells. To this day, there are still far too many licensed medicines routinely prescribed to women day in, day out, with little or no data to support their risks or benefits to womankind. What a scandal!

Along with a lack of evidence for the way medicines work in women, there's also a devastatingly long delay for diagnosis and help with many of the commonest conditions affecting us. Take endometriosis as an example, a disease affecting one in ten women in the UK. One survey found that 50 per cent of all women with endometriosis waited an astonishing six years before finally reaching a diagnosis of this chronic and dreadfully painful gynaecological disorder. Many women reported that they were not satisfied with their practitioner's ability to listen to concerns and felt that their treatment recommendations did not meet their needs.

The gender health gap is real and, although women tend to live longer than men, there are some disturbing trends. For females aged 65 in England, life expectancy increased one year every six years compared to one year every five years for men in the period 2000–2015. Additionally, from 2010 to 2015 life expectancy at age 65 slowed to a one-year increase every 16 years for women and every 9 years for men. Women's healthcare outcomes as we age are trending downwards – and getting worse. Since 2002, the rates of dementia and Alzheimer's among women aged 85 and over have been rising. In particular, from 2002 to 2015 there was a staggering increase of around 175 per cent in dementia as the cause of death in women aged 85, and evidence suggests that women with dementia have fewer visits to the GP, receive less health monitoring and take more potentially harmful medication than men with dementia. Women have also been found to be at particular risk of staying on antipsychotic or sedative medication for longer, probably due to the lower number of appointments where their treatment can be reviewed.

Herein lies one of the fundamental issues we have with our healthcare systems: women are brought up not to complain, to accept that pain – from periods to childbirth and beyond – is part and parcel of being born female. Culturally, we're brought up not to 'waste the doctor's time' with what some might dismiss as worrisome niggles, which our male counterparts might accept far less willingly. Women's health also tends not to be prioritised at a local level, i.e. with your GP. Women respond to pain differently from men – unfortunately, we tend to have more of it, thanks to differences in our nervous systems, sex hormones such as oestrogen and the way our brains behave. Uniquely female problems, such as endometriosis, polycystic ovary syndrome (PCOS), premenstrual syndrome (PMS), vaginal infections, recurrent urinary tract infections (UTIs) and menopause, are too often dismissed as 'just part of being a woman'. Can you imagine men being told that their chronic and debilitating pain condition or scrotum so sore that they can't sit down is 'just part of being a man, so man-up, mate'?

How not to fail

Life coaches often say that the reason most new year's resolutions fail is that we set the bar way too high – that annual mantra of 'I'm going to give up sugar/alcohol/coffee', 'I'm going to stop biting my nails', 'I'm going to shrink by two dress sizes' and so on, all in one go – then we wonder why we fail, feel bad, give up and sink back into our long-established patterns of comfort-zone behaviour (our comfort zone being a very dangerous place to dwell). A more positive outcome happens when we make small habitual changes along the way, incremental benefits that add up over time to long-lasting and game-changing progress.

When you do have a down day, as of course you will, the key is to get back up again. Shake off the negativity dust and congratulate yourself that you're still here, willing and able to get back on track. Talk kindly to yourself, just as you would speak to a friend going through the same process. Acknowledge that you're doing your best in difficult circumstances and pat yourself on the back a bit. No one lives the 'perfect' life. This isn't Instagram; this is reality. The important part is progress, however slow, not perfection. The sole goal is to re-establish the most important relationship you'll ever have in your life – the one you have with yourself.

Stand Up for Your Health

When looking at our own health, both now and going forward, it's important to remember that we're not supposed to have aches and pains. These are early warning signs of something not being right, of things going awry that need fixing before they develop into something more severe. Daily, debilitating symptoms need sorting out, before they escalate. Don't be afraid or hesitant to visit your doctor to discuss health concerns. The sooner they are addressed, the more quickly, easily and cheaply they can be resolved. Educate yourself before making an appointment with your GP, gen up with all the information you can find online and find trusted experts (use reliable sources – you'll find some of the ones I most regularly go to at the back of this book). Write a list of what's happening to you, keep a diary of the changes you've experienced and don't be fobbed off with a prescription for antidepressants or a clinical diagnosis of 'it's just your age'. That's lazy doctoring and you deserve better than that.

Be aware that some GPs may not be fully up to speed on nutritional deficiencies or the safety of modern hormone replacement therapy (HRT), to name a couple of helpful midlife strategies. This is not to shame our medical practitioners, but it's a fact that many are simply not taught about these things at medical school and have so much to cover in their daily practice that they may not be as current in their knowledge as we might hope. Ultimately, who knows more about an illness? The patient who has lived with it for many years, read every book and medical research paper on it, or a medic who attended a single lecture on the subject many years ago? Don't forget that when you have these discussions – *you* are the best person to know what it feels like to live inside your body, even if you don't know why something is happening. That's not to say be confrontational or difficult (most women aren't, despite a tendency or fear of being labelled as such).

Before making a doctor's appointment, ask to see a GP who specialises in women's health. That's a good start and all UK surgeries should have at least one on their books. Go into your appointment feeling calm and confident, armed with factual, evidence-based information and ask for dialogue. Take someone with you if you feel nervous and do take copies of reports and studies if these are helpful to leave for when the doctor has a bit more time to study (and I don't mean a cutting from a tabloid newspaper, justifiably likely to trigger a medical eye roll). Make a list of your symptoms, times, dates and any patterns. Keep in mind the concepts of informed consent and shared decision-making. Here in the UK, the National Institute for Health and Care Excellence (NICE) has published guidelines for all GPs on this. Entitled 'Shared Decision Making', it states that, 'shared decision making for treatment is a joint process in which a healthcare professional works together with a person to reach a decision about care ... based both on evidence and on the person's individual preferences, beliefs and values'. It's your body; it should be your choice as to how it is treated.

If things don't go as well as you would have hoped, don't be afraid to get a second opinion from another doctor at the same surgery. Doctors are human too and opinions, clinical practice and expertise vary. It's always worth reading up on the NICE guidelines for the treatment of any condition too, to check on what is considered to be standard treatment and care.

It's truly never too late to change and make a difference to how you look and feel. Remember, self-care is not self-ish, and it's time now to put yourself at the head of the queue.

Watch out for signs of fluctuating hormones as these impact mood, energy levels, sleep and more. If you're seeing signs of change, ask to see a GP at your surgery specifically trained in women's health (especially menopause care).

This book encourages you to adopt some simple health habits, such as tapping into your circadian rhythm with early-morning sunshine and walking barefoot on the grass whenever you can. These simple, small bio-hacks will make a big difference.

Healthy hacks
- Prioritise YOU! Move your health and wellbeing up your daily to-do list.
- Build in some daily downtime, even if only a few minutes, to take stock of how you're feeling and what simple health hacks you can add in to make yourself feel better.
- Remember that it's not a race – slow and steady wins the day. Consistency is key and even small wins in the day add up to positive progress!

CHAPTER 2

Reversing Ageing with Science

At the age of 60, I'm halfway through my life. That's assuming I make it to 100 or so, like my grandmother and great-grandmother before me. How is this halfway? OK, so I'm not great at maths, but hear me out: the first 20 years or so of all our lives are spent as children growing up and becoming who we are. We go to school, maybe college or university and then we leave home. It is then that life really begins for most of us as independent adults, living on our own terms. I've spent 40 or so years as a functioning adult and, at the age of 60, I would hope to have at least 40 more ahead of me now – hence me being halfway through my life, at the time of writing. Actually, I believe this long-lived age could stretch out much further, given what we're now discovering about longevity, immune function, chrono-ageing and bio-hacking (all of which I'll be covering). A lifespan of 120 years or more could well become the norm – and is something I'm genuinely aiming for.

Many of the functional medicine doctors I speak to boldly state that they're also looking to live until they're at least 120 years old (barring falling under the proverbial bus) and I'm inspired to do likewise. Some, such as a 'father of bio-hacking' Dave Asprey, are on record as saying they're pitching for 180! With the rapid advances in what we know about ageing (and how to hack it) I wouldn't be at all surprised if this were the case. And we can certainly increase our longevity to some extent if we get it right during our middle years. After all, it wasn't that long ago that living past our forties was considered 'well aged'. But if I can speak frankly, what's the point in adding years to our lives if we can't have much life in those years? To quote Mr Spock, it's only really worth it if we can 'live long and prosper', in every sense.

Tapping into Your Longevity

A few years ago, in my mid-fifties, I had my biological markers of age tested (physical fitness, muscle mass, blood markers, telomere length – part of our DNA that gets shorter as we age, see box below – and so on) which showed my biological age to be 39. It's gone up a bit since then (I'm currently at 45), having lived through the stress of divorce, lockdowns, selling my farm, building businesses, parenting teens and navigating a major house move, but I intend to reduce my biological age back down again over the next few years with my stack of healthy pro-ageing habits.

Instead of growing older and less capable, I'm pushing the clock back to become ever more able, physically, mentally and emotionally.

We're lucky enough to be living in an era where biometric testing is becoming more mainstream, where we can track everything from our glucose response to deep sleep brain waves and more with wearable fitness gadgets. We can take simple DNA cheek-swab tests to see how we process certain nutrients or what genetic variances might be influencing our susceptibility to diseases. Pin-prick blood tests give us a snapshot of hormone balance, blood fats and vitamin levels, while poo swabs can pick up a microbiome in need of rebalancing.

Tapping into our longevity with ways to live and age well is no longer the preserve of Silicon Valley hi-tech billionaire bio-hackers with their personal cryo-chambers and daily IV vitamin drip infusions. Nor is it confined to the super-fit gym bunnies or hypermobile yogis, living on diets of spirulina smoothies and daily spin classes. While some tests are still quite pricey, useful finger-prick tests for blood fats, vitamin D and so on can often be found in chemists and online at a lower cost.

> **Telomere length**
> Telomere shortening has been discovered to be a primary metric of ageing and age-related diseases including cancer, autoimmune issues and heart disease. Finding ways to preserve our telomere length has become something of an obsession within certain longevity science circles, with Telomere Length Analysis being seen as a potentially useful index of biological versus chronological age.

The Science of Genomics

Think of your genes as a deck of cards: you've been dealt a hand at birth. You may not hold the best cards, but it's how well you play them that determines how long you stay in the game (ask any poker player). This playing of our 'deck of cards' is essentially the science of genomics. Nutrigenomics, a specialist branch of genomics, is all about the modifications we can make to our DNA that will switch certain genes 'on' or 'off', depending on a variety of diet and lifestyle factors. It's the process by which we can identify our strengths and weaknesses as determined by our DNA – and act accordingly. Play your cards right, and chances are greatly improved for living a longer, happier life.

The modern science of nutrigenomics is advancing at speed and is a fast-moving, exciting field of medicine worth learning a bit more about. Previously undiscovered bits of the human genome are being unravelled all the time, revealing new protocols for gene expression, meaning how our genes vary from person to person. These genetic variances are called single nucleotide polymorphisms, referred to as SNPs (pronounced 'snips') for short. Various genomic variants found within our DNA have been identified as impacting a mass of physiological and psychological functions. For example, how sensitive we are to caffeine comes down to two particular genes: CYP1A2 (responsible for the way we process and detoxify caffeine) and ADORA2A (a receptor gene responsible for how sensitive we are to caffeine).

Here's the science for those interested in a deep dive into gene expression: caffeine is metabolised in the liver by the cytochrome P450 oxidase enzyme system. CYP1A2 is the main deactivator (detoxifier) of caffeine. Variants on this gene increase its activity so it is metabolised more quickly, reducing the duration of effect. Then there's adenosine, a by-product of energy release, which interacts with the ADORA2A receptor gene to inhibit dopamine. This is a reason why some of us feel more tired after exercise and later in the day. Caffeine inhibits ADORA2A, which frees up dopamine to exert its stimulatory effects. ADORA2A genetic variants increase sensitivity to caffeine, which means that all those with this genetic SNP will find that a small amount of caffeine can have a significant stimulatory effect.

You may not need a genetic test to discover this gene variance (although I've listed a few of my favourite testing resources at the back of the book if you're curious to seek confirmation – see page 307). If this is you, you'll be more sensitive to the stimulating effects of caffeine, identified by feeling jittery after a single cup of coffee. Others may find that they can develop a tolerance for caffeine, but may be more likely to become coffee addicts, craving that cup of strong coffee to get the day started. This is due to the expression of this gene, meaning you react more than most to the uplifting and stimulating effects of caffeine, so your body unconsciously craves its effects. This is not necessarily a bad thing, as coffee has been shown to have many health benefits (detailed on page 191), but ideally, those who feel the pull towards their morning espresso (I include myself here) would also possess the genes that enable their cells to easily process caffeine out of their systems, in this case a fast CYP1A2 gene. If they don't, their bodies are likely to be left feeling jarred and jittery, unable to properly process the more stimulating effects of coffee, leading to anxiety, nervous tension and disrupted sleep – all of which can influence mental health and physical longevity.

My own nutrigenomic DNA tests revealed that I have a strong response to caffeine (which is why I do so love my morning flat-white fix) but that I also have a version of the CYP1A2 gene that processes it slightly more slowly. Armed with this knowledge, I now try not to drink caffeine after 2pm, so my body has time to process it out of my system well before bedtime.

This is just one example of how gene variations influence our daily lives and how having a better understanding of our genetic make-up can enable us to shortcut or 'hack' our way to better health. In the future, we're likely to be able to ask our doctors for a routine set of genetic tests that will give us the clues we need to live better, according to our individual health risks and requirements. We're going to be able to discover risk factors for degenerative diseases, sensitivity to alcohol, sugars, inflammation, gut disorders and cognitive decline, as well as reveal how well we process nutrients such as vitamin D or foods such as lactose and gluten – all tests that are available to us now at a price, but which in the future will become the norm, possibly even a blueprint that can be obtained at birth.

Blood tests and microbiome analysis can also provide us with another form of testing. These provide a snapshot of our vitamin and hormone status and can be very helpful in guiding our supplement and replacement hormone choices. However, keep in mind that these can only give an indication of our status on the day they are taken, and can fluctuate from one day to the next. This is especially true of hormone tests, as our hormones differ even from one hour to the next. Being guided by our symptoms is a more reliable measure – more on this in Chapter 3 when I take a closer look at our hormonal health.

Sometimes, it makes sense for a blood test to be carried out alongside a genetic screen to assess gene response. For example, you might find you have plenty of vitamin D, well within the 'normal' range, but if you don't have the genetics to utilise it, you'll likely need to take more to bring your own body up to the levels it needs for optimum health. This is one reason why I am personally such a fan of genetic testing – and gave all those in my immediate family a testing kit of their own one Christmas; possibly the best gift I've ever given, as it helped identify and sort out several long-standing health issues.

This is a fascinating and exciting time to be connected with the world of wellbeing.

Never before has so much information and inside knowledge of our own bodily systems been available to us as individuals.

Together with judicious and responsible use of the internet (a resource to be treated with extreme caution when it comes to healthcare) we have an amazing opportunity to make the very best choices for fitness, diet, lifestyle and so much more. With advances in modern medicine (surgery, scans, diagnostic testing for bespoke prescribed medication) we may well be looking forward to literally doubling the 'three score years and ten' lifespan often quoted from Biblical and Shakespearean texts. What an extraordinary and exciting thought.

How to Increase Your Odds with Bio-hacking

Alongside genetic predisposition, the latest nutritional research is revealing more than ever before about the working of our bodies at a cellular level and the ways this influences how well we age. This is the geeky bit of longevity science that lights my fire more than I can say, so buckle up and enjoy some of the highlights and headlines about how to thrive in older age:

Sirtuins

Sirtuins are a family of genes, which code for proteins, and are involved in cellular health, including SIRT2 that regulates inflammation and SIRT6 linked to longer lifespan. Fundamentally important when it comes to how well we age, they're exciting longevity scientists because they help regulate our gene expression. By supporting our sirtuin activity, we're enhancing our ability to increase our life-/healthspan by protecting and repairing DNA. Sirtuins are considered important in the prevention of cancer, as they help detect when a cell is cancerous and suppress its replication (we make cancer cells all the time; the problem occurs when they multiply out of control). Sirtuins also protect our heart and cardiovascular function by reducing oxidative stress (when free radicals get too active and push our antioxidants out of balance in the body) and improving blood pressure (see also page 131 for five easy ways to lower your blood pressure). They regulate glucose and fat metabolism, and help cognitive function by improving memory, reducing neuroinflammation and guarding against age-related brain function decline. As if this isn't enough, sirtuins also help protect against and heal inflammation, the root cause of so many diseases and autoimmune conditions. We're going to hear far more about sirtuins in the coming years, specifically ways in which we can help support sirtuin activity for a longer, healthier life. So get used to this word. The message is simple: look after your sirtuins and they will look after you. Sirtuins are fussy critters though and will only do their job well if they're given nicotinamide adenine dinucleotide (NAD+) to get them going.

NAD+

This is a naturally occurring co-enzyme (form of niacin, vitamin B3) found in every cell of our bodies and is broadly used to help protect and energise cells. It helps to convert nutrients from our food into energy for our bodies. Another of its crucial roles though is to 'feed' our sirtuins so that they can do their job repairing damaged DNA and improving our energy production. Unfortunately for us, our NAD+ supplies reduce as we age (levels in the body actually halve every 20 years from birth) which is bad news because we really do need this co-enzyme for all forms of cellular energy, including sirtuin activity. So the connection between sirtuins, NAD+ and how well and healthily we age is fundamental.

Although we produce less NAD+ as we get older, our bodies' demand for it actually increases as we use it to fight rising levels of inflammation, stress, environmental pollutants and the like. NAD+ acts as fuel for the sirtuins; without it, sirtuins simply can't function – and there are strategies to support this that I'm going to come back to many times during the next few chapters.

Some of the simplest ways to increase our NAD+ is by putting the body under a bit of acute stress. This might be a 60-second blast in an ice-cold shower (this is the science-y bit as to why that health hack works), a few minutes of intense (HIIT) exercise (see my own 10-minute HIIT regime on pages 245–249), eating polyphenols or spices (such as chilli or ginger), drinking green tea (the active ingredient is epigallocatechin gallate (EGCG)) and intermittent fasting (for example, some kind of calorie restriction – see page 174). Foods high in niacin (vitamin B3) such as liver, chicken breast, pork, beef, peanuts, avocado, brown rice and peas provide natural precursors to NAD+. We can also take a daily supplement to support NAD+, which, of course, is the easiest and most foolproof way to ensure consistent supplies. NAD+ supplements don't actually contain NAD+ itself though – they're made with its precursors or molecules that give the body the building blocks to make NAD+. Two of the commonly promoted precursors for NAD+ are NMN (which we met earlier – see page 35) and nicotinamide riboside (NR). These are the building blocks for NAD+, shown to be effective at improving overall NAD+ levels in the body.

As you read in my morning routine section on page 35, I take a small scoop of NMN every morning under my tongue (I also take a cold shower to enhance its effect). I'll talk more about the differences between NR and NMN on page 290 when looking at longevity supplements in more detail. Other NAD+ promoters include the potent antioxidants alpha-lipoic acid resveratrol, curcumin (from turmeric) and quercetin (one of my personal favourites as it also dramatically reduces allergy and hay fever symptoms). If you'd like to add these in too you'll find more on pages 289, 69 and 251.

Zombie cells

On the other side of the coin to sirtuins, we find senescent, or 'zombie', cells. Just as sirtuins can help promote youthfulness and longevity, so zombie cells can accelerate the ageing process.

All of our cells have a natural lifecycle: they are born, they divide, multiply and die, moving on to be recycled by the body. However, there is another form of cell death called apoptosis, which differs from this pattern and may not be uniform across all cell types. All cells suffer damage that causes them to mutate or die, from factors such as alcohol, smoking, pesticides and other environmental pollutants, together with stress, disease and lack of sleep, to name a few. However, as we get older, some cells are better able to divide and renew than others. We accumulate more ageing cells as we get older, referred to by those studying longevity as an increased amount of 'cellular senescence'. This is when we have a greater number of decrepit old cells that hang around in the body, a bit like the living dead (hence their nickname 'zombie' cells), damaging other cells and disturbing cellular systems. It may amaze you to learn that around 1 million cells die in our bodies each and every *second*, becoming replenished with fresh, young cells. But as with everything else in the body, this process slows down with age. So not only do we make fewer healthy new cells, the old and defunct ones tend to hang around for longer too.

Zombie cells, or senescent cells, no longer multiply but they don't completely die off either. Instead, they release malevolent molecules that spark inflammation. The immune system is pretty good at picking up these senescent cells, but it becomes less efficient at doing so as we age. Senescent cells tend to build up, driving more inflammation and potentially leading to degenerative diseases such as Alzheimer's, certain cancers and osteoarthritis. That's not to say senescent or zombie cells are all bad. One study carried out at the University of California, published in the journal *Science* in October 2022, showed they can help repair lung tissue damage by encouraging stem cells to grow, so there may be a case for senescent cells being part of the wound-healing process. As with everything, it's about finding the right balance within the body. Shutting down the negative effects of too many senescent cells (which we'll explore on the next page), while also allowing some of their potential benefits to remain active, is something researchers are still trying to unpick.

Autophagy

One of the best ways to clear out an unhealthy overload of zombie cells is with a natural internal clean-up process called autophagy, which literally means self-eating. Sounds a bit too close to our zombie discussion for comfort? Well, self-eating is actually good for our overall health, especially when it comes to longevity. Think of it as the ultimate form of bio-recycling. The body breaks down and reuses old, redundant cell parts so our cells can work more effectively. We literally eat ourselves clean to survive. Autophagy is a form of essential spring cleaning, but as we've seen with so many biochemical activities, it's something that also decreases with age, leading to a greater build-up of cellular junk that could really do with clearing out.

The body produces a large amount of dead and damaged cell material every second of our lives. Unseen and unaware, it's not good to have a build-up of this hanging around our systems, especially as we age. Depending on how hard we've lived (or partied!) these past few decades, we're likely to have accumulated a whole heap of toxic cell debris inside us. The purpose of autophagy is to remove this cellular rubbish and get the body back on track, so it can function in a healthier, fresher, younger state. Getting into a state of autophagy is a bit like running a defrag programme on your computer, seeking out the damaged bits of cellular clutter and literally devouring them, ridding the body of them. Autophagy can also be used to help break the cycle of metabolic and autoimmune disorders, as it forces the body to take a break from the way it usually operates, making it run on an entirely different mode – it's a bit like downloading an entirely new operating system, to continue with the computer analogy.

When the body is in a state of autophagy, it starts by cleaning up waste material from cells as a form of fuel for the body (literally self-eating for energy and survival). Having mopped up much of the toxic debris, it then looks around to see what else it can 'eat' and heads for our stored fat deposits, eating into these. This is why prolonged periods of fasting (or putting the body into a state of ketosis – more about this on page 132) can be so effective at losing those hard-to-shift excess pounds that don't seem to respond to conventional calorie restriction. Autophagy also has an effect on hormones involved in weight regulation, including glucagon, insulin and ghrelin (the hunger hormone) and may also play a role in fat metabolism, increasing lipolysis, which is the breakdown of fat droplets so they can be excreted from the body.

> **Autophagy is a vitally important process we need to be more aware of if we want to give our bodies the best chance of living well for longer.**

Although autophagy is a natural process, it's triggered by somehow stressing our cells to get them to switch into survival mode. Here are four ways we can do that:

Fasting

It's not known exactly how long we need to go without food to trigger autophagy, but it seems to start after around 24–48 hours, and be best around 72 hours. At the Buchinger Wilhelmi clinics in Germany and Spain (run by the Wilhelmi family of doctors, the founding fathers of fasting), they advocate a five-day fasting protocol involving 500Kcal of juice or broths a day, together with colon cleanses. I'll cover this in more detail on page 203 (see also Useful Resources on page 305).

Calorie restriction
Instead of depriving the body of food (fasting), we can trigger autophagy by decreasing the amount of energy available to the body to use (calories), forcing our cells into autophagy to compensate for the lack of food as fuel.

High-fat, low-carb diet
Also known as keto, this changes the way the body burns energy, switching from sugars (glucose) to using fats (ketones) for fuel. This switch can trigger autophagy, but it is very specific. To get into a state of ketosis, virtually any kinds of sugars (including those found in whole grains, fruits and vegetables) are off-limits.

Exercise
Provided it's high intensity, a short burst of vigorous exercise has been shown to be sufficient to trigger autophagy. Admittedly, the study that proved this was carried out using mice on a treadmill . . . but the theory is sound.

Autophagy is definitely something to be aware of when it comes to improving longevity and healthspan. Beloved by bio-hackers, it's also gaining a lot of attention within the mainstream medical community for its potential in preventing or even treating cancer, as well as serious neurodegenerative diseases such as Parkinson's and Alzheimer's. Although in its infancy, some studies suggest that many cancerous cells can be removed by putting the body into a state of autophagy. Ongoing research at the Buchingher Wilhelmi fasting clinics in Germany and Spain is also showing that just one five-day fasting-induced period of autophagy (under medical supervision) can help prevent migraine attacks from reoccurring in those who are regularly affected. It was certainly one of the things that helped my eldest daughter, Lily.

How to cheat at autophagy

If you're intrigued to try autophagy but not keen on the idea of exhausting yourself on a treadmill, turning to keto or fasting for five days straight, one shortcut to consider is the food supplement spermidine. This natural substance is a polyamine – a dietary molecule found in certain foods that interacts with our DNA. Linked to cell ageing, spermidine mimics the effects of autophagy in the body.

The richest natural sources of spermidine are natto (a mushy mix of extremely pungent fermented soya beans, an acquired taste, popular in Japan), cheese, wheatgerm and chlorella. A diet naturally rich in spermidine is probably a key reason why those living in Okinawa, Japan, are so very long-lived, with a high proportion of locals living well past 100 years and more. One of the longest-lived populations in the world, the average life expectancy for women in Okinawa is over 90 years old. To demonstrate the power of natto, a 2021 study reported in the journal *Medical Sciences* found that feeding 45–90g of natto daily to healthy male volunteers for one year resulted in lower pro-inflammatory markers, with dietary spermidine shown to cross the blood–brain barrier, potentially reducing neurodegeneration.

While researchers are still exploring the precise mechanisms for how spermidine works, studies show that taking supplements of it can induce autophagy. This may not be the same as, say, a five-day fast, but a combination of approaches could be beneficial, possibly reducing fasting time to as little as two or three days. Supplementing with spermidine seems to improve many of the hallmarks of ageing, from stem cell exhaustion, muscle cell regeneration, DNA protection and repairs to damaged DNA within hair follicles (potentially useful for anyone concerned about age-related hair loss). Spermidine supplementation also seems to improve insulin signalling and preserve telomere length, a sign of how well we're ageing – the longer our telomeres, the better. Spermidine (and autophagy itself) also improves mitochondrial function (our cellular energy processes), which declines with age. Mitochondria dysfunction can accelerate ageing by reducing cell energy, increasing inflammatory processes and activating cell death pathways – all pretty scary-sounding stuff. Spermidine has been shown to mitigate this, as well as playing a role in suppressing cell senescence (back to those terror zombie cells again).

Writing a review of data in the journal *Aging Science* in December 2022, a team of research professors concluded: 'Spermidine supplementation elongates the healthspan and lifespan of multiple species ... elevated dietary intake alleviates, delays or halts age-associated deteriorations, including cancer, cardiovascular disease and cognitive dysfunction'. It doesn't get much more definitive than that from a team of clinical researchers. Although one of the newer supplements on the market, research suggests that spermidine has many benefits and no known adverse effects, so it is something I now take daily (see page 183).

Our Mighty Mitochondria

In a nutshell, mitochondria are parts of cells that generate most of the energy needed to power cellular activity. They're involved in the production of adenosine triphosphate (ATP), the main molecule used by our cells for energy. Without ATP, the body can't function. Without healthy mitochondrial activity, we can't make sufficient ATP for our bodies' needs. In essence, mitochondria are our bodies' batteries.

Tiny, but mighty, viewed under the microscope, mitochondria are tiny 'shell' shapes containing ribosomes (which produce protein), mitochondrial DNA and a matrix of fluids rich in enzymes and proteins. These enzymes are especially significant when it comes to creating ATP molecules for energy. This is a monumentally massive task – a healthy person will probably produce around their entire body weight of ATP every day! This is a phenomenal feat and needs to happen because the body can't store ATP, so it needs to be made on a continuous basis, each and every second of the day (and night). The production of ATP is so important that it takes up around 25 per cent of our cells' volume, with most of the ATP produced being used in the brain, which is why there is such a strong connection between mitochondrial dysfunction and neurodegeneration or brain disease.

In addition to making energy, mitochondria also detoxify ammonia in our liver cells and play an important role in apoptosis, the death of cells we discussed earlier. They're also important for building blood cells and various hormones, including oestrogen and testosterone – more of which for midlife women in the next chapter! They determine how healthy our cells are. When our mitochondria fail, our organs fail – and we fail.

REVERSING AGEING WITH SCIENCE

So, how do we ensure our mitochondria are supported and do not fail us? That is one of the most important questions when it comes to living and ageing well. Firstly, genetics do play a part. We may have been blessed with a strong genetic predisposition to mitochondrial health – or less so. How do you know? Well, instinctively, you may know you're someone with a lowered immune system, as you're always the one catching flu bugs or you don't feel as physically strong or as intrinsically robust as others. For a more precise diagnosis, there are various genetic marker tests you can do if you're curious, but my view is to assume your mitochondria need all the support you can give them – that way you can't fail but feel better for it. This is especially important as we age, as once we reach around 55 years of age, our mitochondrial damage starts to accumulate and we may feel that we're literally running out of steam. If this is you, be aware of what is happening right now, but also be encouraged that there's plenty you can do about it. In a brilliant article entitled 'Mitochondria – Fundamental to Life and Health', Dr Joseph Pizzorno, editor in chief of *Integrative Medicine: A Clinician's Journal* wrote, 'With such a long list of common diseases . . . early ageing, Alzheimer's, autism, cardiovascular disease, dementia, diabetes, migraine, Parkinson's disease . . . caused by or aggravated by mitochondrial dysfunction, it is difficult to overstate its importance'.

So how best to support our minuscule but mighty powerhouses of ATP production? Much like the rest of the body, our mitochondria rely on nutrients for fuel and are damaged by the usual lifestyle suspects: environmental pollutants, alcohol, heavy metals (such as mercury from deep sea fish and dental fillings), many prescription and non-prescription drugs (antibiotics, statins, aspirin and ibuprofen, to name just a few) and oxidative damage (such as stress). Quite a few varied nutrients are needed for mitochondrial activity, but a few stand out as being key. These are the B-complex vitamins – notably B1, B2, B3, riboflavin, co-enzyme Q10 (CoQ10), carnitine, iron, magnesium, manganese and cysteine (glutathione). Several of these nutrients are already well known to us, but below are a few useful nuggets of information on a couple that are perhaps less well known.

How to minimise mitochondrial stress

Reduce your exposure to environmental pollutants as much as possible. Don't smoke (or vape) and avoid smoky environments. If an atmosphere smells bad, it probably is bad! That includes dry cleaners and nail bars without adequate ventilation. Avoid using aerosol sprays (such as fabric protectants or insecticides) in confined spaces and don't breathe in the fumes from household cleaning agents.

Co-enzyme Q10

Dubbed the 'energy nutrient' for good reason, CoQ10 is vital for healthy mitochondria and, therefore, ATP (energy) production. It's found in most tissues in the body, especially the heart, kidneys, liver and muscles. It's an antioxidant, so helps neutralise the destructive effects of free radical cell damage, and studies have claimed it to be the only nutrient showing therapeutic benefits for those with severe mitochondrial disorders. It has also been shown to alter gene expression (in mice) which is encouraging as mice share much of our physiology, anatomy and metabolism, which is why they're so widely used in medical research before human trials. Since the genome sequence of a mouse was published back in 2002, we know that we share many of the same traits, making genetic research using mice even more valuable for humans. Mice and humankind have many of the same genes responsible for degenerative diseases linked to ageing, such as atherosclerosis (the build-up of plaque in the arteries) and hypertension (high blood pressure). A mouse also has a much shorter lifespan – typically one mouse year equals 30 human years, making it much faster to measure the effects of ageing in mice than in humans.

Studies (in both humans as well as mice) looking at the activity of CoQ10 supplementation on our mitochondria have thrown up some interesting findings. One notable benefit has been shown for reducing muscle pain experienced by those taking statins, as well as for those with general muscle pain and weakness (often genetic). (Other ways to help reduce muscle stiffness include gentle exercise, such as yoga, and taking magnesium, omega-3, hyaluronic acid and collagen supplements, which can also be very helpful, alongside HRT for those with lowered oestrogen supplies.) It should be noted that statins reduce our CoQ10 levels, so if you are taking these drugs you should firstly do some independent research as to whether they're really necessary for your own individual needs and, if the answer is clearly yes, consider taking a daily supplement of CoQ10 (I have included a helpful book on statins in the Useful Resources, page 309). Other studies investigating treatments for Parkinson's disease have also shown benefits, with CoQ10 supplements of up to 3,000mg daily shown to slow the progression of the disease and be both beneficial and safe. Overall, we become less efficient at processing CoQ10 as we age, which reduces our mitochondrial activity, so finding ways to better support this as we get older can only be a good thing. Eating foods such as oily fish and organ meats (such as liver) also helps boost our supplies without supplementation. Lesser supplies are also found in plant-based sources, such as nuts, seeds and soya beans.

Glutathione

I've become much more aware in recent years of this interesting nutrient, dubbed the 'master antioxidant'. It's one of the most important molecules we need to live and age well and, for something so important, I'm surprised it's not more of a buzzword – or that it took me so long to discover it. Our bodies make glutathione naturally in the liver from the amino acids glycine, cysteine and glutamic acid (one reason why it's important to eat plenty of protein-rich foods, which we'll further explore in Chapter 4). Not only is it vital for mitochondrial health, glutathione is also linked to NAD+, helps build and repair tissues, working alongside other antioxidants to keep them in balance, and supports protein synthesis and the immune system. Low glutathione levels have been linked with cancer, type 2 diabetes, hepatitis and HIV/AIDS. It's a vital part of maintaining our mitochondrial activity and strengthens our overall mitochondrial DNA. So, that's pretty important you'd agree?

Unfortunately – yet again – our supplies dwindle as we age and we become less efficient at making glutathione. To compound this deficit, up to a third of us actually lack the gene expressions needed to convert the amino acids required into glutathione. This means we simply don't make it – or we don't make it very well. This was something I discovered for myself when I did a simple nutrigenomic DNA test. I was surprised to learn that I simply don't have the GSTM1 gene needed for my body to convert nutrients from food into glutathione. That was a bit of a shock, to be honest. How had I (and others like me) survived so well for so long without this basic ability? Well, it was probably down to other supportive genetic and environmental factors, together with the fact that eating a wide range of many other helpful antioxidants, such as vitamins C and E, for so many years now has been my mainstay. But I have to say, once armed with this knowledge, I rushed out the same day and bought myself some glutathione supplements. I took one capsule that evening and woke up with tangibly renewed energy. I actually felt as though someone had reached inside me and replaced my ageing batteries with a brand new set. I've taken glutathione most evenings ever since. As the lack of glutathione-creating genes is so common, I'd advise anyone lacking in energy to try a supplement. You don't necessarily need a genetic test to tell you if it works – after a few days you may feel renewed, or not. However, a deficiency is not always immediately obvious, so a supplement would probably be prudent for all mid-lifers.

One last little gem of information on glutathione: it has been shown to neutralise hydrogen peroxide (think greying hair!) and there have been a few clinical studies showing those with low blood levels of glutathione to be more susceptible to going grey. As our loss of melanin is linked to oxidative stress, there may be some kind of genetic pathway for glutathione that is involved. It has also been shown to even out pigmentation on the skin (in South Asia, glutathione supplements are popular for lightening the skin). I have not seen direct evidence for skin lightening, but a more even, brighter skin tone is often seen by those who take glutathione, especially for areas of sun-damaged skin. Whether for health, longevity or beauty, the data definitely supports glutathione supplementation as we age.

Glutathione is a fussy substance though, as it gets broken down by the acids and enzymes in the stomach before it can reach the liver, so taking the usual tablet form of supplements is not a very effective way to top up our supplies. Bio-hackers tend to favour IV-glutathione delivered via a drip in a clinic for an instant 'hit' of energy, but these are time-consuming, expensive and not very practical for everyday life. I think liposomal delivery systems are a good option, where molecules of a nutrient such as glutathione are encased in protective fatty 'bubbles', small enough to be absorbed directly into our cells, bypassing the stomach altogether. Liposomes make it easy for whatever has been put inside them to slip inside our cells for maximum absorption and availability. I take my glutathione in liposomal form, either as a capsule, gel or liquid (I've listed the brands I buy on page 313). I mostly take it in the evening and find it very helpful for giving me extra energy, as well as reducing the effects of alcohol the following morning, if I've been drinking. Unfortunately, because liposomal technology is expensive, these supplements do tend to be quite pricey. They're also susceptible to fraud and there have been court cases brought against some supplement suppliers claiming to sell liposomal supplements when, in fact, none was detected after testing. Never buy on price alone. Always check independent and verified reviews and read up on the independent testing process and quality control on a brand's website before buying. One way to tell whether or not your supplement is truly liposomal is to pop it in some water. Genuine liposomes do not dissolve (they're fat-soluble, not water-soluble), so will swirl around in a mass of gel-like globules in a glass of water. If taking glutathione, it's worth also topping up with zinc too, ensuring a daily supply of at least around 30mg, as glutathione can lower zinc levels.

For the majority who are able to make glutathione from the amino acid building blocks found in protein-rich foods, you may not need to take a supplement as long as you're giving your body enough of the basics it needs to make its own (see page 138).

Alongside the amino acids glycine, cysteine and glutamic acid, a number of other interesting food supplements help support the making of glutathione, including curcumin (from turmeric), N-acetylcysteine (NAC), selenium, silymarin (milk thistle extract – possibly the reason why this herb is so helpful for liver detoxing), vitamins C and E. We can also find small amounts of glutathione itself in some foods, especially cruciferous vegetables (the ones that taste slightly bitter due to their sulphur compounds) such as cabbage, broccoli, cauliflower, Brussels sprouts and watercress, and alliums, such as leeks, onions and garlic. It's also found in unprocessed meat, asparagus, avocados and spinach, although when eaten it does tend to be broken down in the stomach before it can be used by the liver. One tip is to crush or chop these kinds of veggies (especially garlic) to help release their bioactive glucosinolate molecules before they hit the stomach, and only ever lightly cook or steam them, or eat them raw.

Selenium also supports glutathione production, so make sure you're eating a little of this too (only very small amounts are needed – **never** take more than is recommended as a daily dose of any supplement, as an overdose can be fatally toxic). A good way to get enough selenium is to eat two Brazil nuts daily (said by the *American Journal of Clinical Nutrition* to be sufficient). Wild-caught fish (notably salmon) and grass-fed beef are also good sources of selenium, or take a supplement that includes its active form, selenomethionine. Exercise and sleep also support our glutathione supplies (so be sure to get quality amounts of both on a regular basis – we'll discuss these two important wellbeing pillars in Chapters 9 and 10).

There are so many ways we can help build better health and optimise our longevity by reducing our exposure to environmental pollutants, feeding our cells with helpful nutrients from specific foods and/or supplements and building more muscle mass. Activities such as lifting weights and strength training have a significant and positive impact on our mitochondria, so I'll talk more about this when discussing how best to exercise in midlife and beyond in Chapter 9.

I hope this chapter has given you an insight into some of the fascinating research ongoing in the world of longevity life sciences. Much of what I've covered forms part of what is termed 'functional medicine'. That is the how and why of what makes illness occur in the body and how we can restore our health by addressing the root cause of diseases – even before they take hold. Functional medicine differs from the 'conventional' kind in that it aims to uncover *why* a problem has occurred and not just fix the symptom of that problem. As a simple example, a conventional medic may prescribe an anti-inflammatory painkiller for an arthritic knee to relieve the agony, whereas a functional medicine medic is more likely to dig deeper into *why the knee has become inflamed and hurts in the first place – and then look at fixing the cause. This is obviously good news, as not only does it prevent a disorder from getting worse and affecting other areas of the body, but it also reduces the need for prescription medication and its many attendant side effects. Don't get me wrong – I'm a massive fan of acute medical care and many of the advances we're making in modern medicine, but I'm an even bigger fan of solving the 'whys?' in the first place. I've listed a few contacts for functional medicine practitioners on page 307, which can be a good place to start if you're interested in doing any of the nutrigenomic or other forms of bio-testing and analysis. These include Glycanage, a well-respected finger prick blood test which gives you your biological age based on levels of inflammation.*

Healthy hacks

- Get your sirtuins on side to improve longevity by eating more protein in your diet and taking up some form of short-burst, high-intensity exercise and consider taking supplements such as NAD+, NMN, alpha-lipoic acid, quercetin and/or resveratrol to enhance their activity.

- Consider taking a CoQ10 supplement, especially once past the age of 50 when we become less efficient at processing it. This is especially important if on any kind of medication that makes you feel tired, notably statins. If you feel tired, suffer from energy slumps and/or muscle aches you'll probably feel better taking a daily dose of CoQ10.

- Boost your daily glutathione supplies by eating more leafy greens, especially cruciferous vegetables. Super-green heroes you should always have to hand include anything from the brassica family, such as broccoli (baby broccoli sprouts are just 'the bomb' to borrow one of my kids' favourite expressions), Brussels sprouts, cabbage (all kinds), collard greens and turnips.

CHAPTER 3

Hormone Hacking

For women in midlife and later years, many of the 'whys?' when it comes to symptoms of ill health are due to shifting hormones, which leads me neatly on to the perimenopause and menopause – two stages in life I've been passionately highlighting for many years now. In fact, I can't write a book about living a better second half without a significant look at our hormones. When I wrote *The Good Menopause Guide* back in 2018, the very word 'menopause' was a no-no, spoken in hushed tones (if at all), associated as it was back then with incontinence and decrepitude. But in the space of a few short, but challenging, years that has mostly changed, thanks in no small part to a few key pioneers, passionately advocating for midlife women's health – like Dr Louise Newson, a truly inspirational woman who continues to be the leading UK educator, tirelessly campaigning for women to have greater access to evidence-based information and better health-care services. I work hard most days, but she makes me look like a slacker. Her net has spread far and wide; founding the free Balance Menopause app (see page 308), a brilliant resource that reaches millions of women around the globe to put safe, trusted information right into their hands. She's also the founder of the

Newson Health Menopause Society, a not-for-profit research organisation (that doesn't accept any funding from the pharmaceutical industry, unlike so many charities and healthcare research organisations) and The Menopause Charity in the UK. I'm very proud to have been this charity's first official ambassador. But despite all this activity and so much more by many others, together with the massive rise in awareness, there are still many menopause myths that persist, which is why I continue to be spurred on by the overwhelming need to talk about the benefits of natural hormones to help improve women's lives.

Before we take a look at hormones and how they can help, hinder or heal us, it's important to say that the menopause is a natural stage in every woman's life, generally occurring when we reach our late forties or early fifties. For some women, it can be much earlier (around 3 in 100 women will experience their menopause as early as in their twenties or thirties). Others may be plunged into a 'surgical menopause' after a hysterectomy, oophorectomy (removal of one or both ovaries) or may become menopausal due to medical treatments such as those for some types of cancers. Too many women find themselves stranded in midlife without their hormones, either as they decline or are medically taken away. Others may be oblivious to the hormone changes happening to their minds and bodies and put their multitude of symptoms down to general declining age, stress or burnout. I put myself in that last category. I had absolutely no idea that my crippling headaches, low mood, anxiety, aching joints, recurrent UTIs – even tinnitus – were not, in fact, caused by the stress I was under both at home and at work, but were a direct consequence of my fluctuating, lowering and, ultimately, lost hormones.

I'd like to make it clear that discussing help for menopausal symptoms is *not* somehow medicalising the menopause. For most, it's about recognising that this is a significant time of life that marks the end of their 'first half', a time of having periods and being able to procreate. For some, it can happen much earlier due to genetics, medical treatment or surgery. It's also about being sufficiently informed to ask the right questions and able to move seamlessly onwards through this inevitable phase in the healthiest way possible.

Instead of fearing 'The Change' and living in dread of its effects, I'd like to reframe this time as one of positivity and midlife empowerment.

This should be when older women can feel more energised than ever before, as they shift into period-free living for the first time in many decades.

Ultimately, we women are ruled by our hormones. That's a biological fact of life thanks to our XX chromosomes. But that can be a positive! I like the expression 'me-no-pause'. This can truly be a time to embrace as it allows us to move forward, free from periods, PMS and child-rearing commitments. No more costly and cumbersome sanitary protection, monthly bloating, risk of unwanted pregnancy, contraception . . . There is so much to celebrate. But as a realist I know that this new-found freedom and sense of joy is a rare reality. For the overwhelming majority of midlife women who contact me (daily, on social media), menopause means misery. So it is my fervent wish that my work in this area will help inform, inspire and empower *all* women to get the help they need. I am 110 per cent driven to provide evidence-based information, knowledge and objectivity for you to equip yourself with the information you need to make the healthcare and support choices that are right for you – and never taking 'no' for an answer when you choose to make informed decisions about your own body and how you would like to be helped.

Be Guided by Your Symptoms

Women's bodies are a mass of hormones, notably oestrogen, found in every cell from brain, to bones and bladder and beyond. Which is why, when our oestrogen levels start to fluctuate and lower in midlife, all kinds of different symptoms are triggered. Some women may claim to have sailed through their menopausal years without so much as a backward glance, but when more closely questioned, will admit to feeling tired, having achy joints or insomnia, anxiety, dry eyes, recurrent UTIs, vaginal dryness, osteoporosis, headaches, low mood, loss of confidence, tiredness, memory loss, hair loss, mood swings and/or potentially more . . . all symptoms and health problems caused or worsened by lowered oestrogen levels, yet not as widely recognised as the more commonly cited night sweats or hot flushes.

Unlike a tap, our hormones don't suddenly switch off one day. Instead, they ebb and flow, fluctuating by the hour in some cases and certainly changing day by day. This is why high-street menopause testing kits are a waste of time and money. At what point do we test ourselves when our hormones vary so wildly? The answer is we can't. The government NICE guidelines are clear on this: blood tests to determine hormone levels for women over the age of 45 should not be carried out because they may well produce a false positive or negative result, leading to an incorrect conclusion and plan of care. In fact, they're generally unreliable and can be misleading at any age.

So if blood tests are not the answer, how do we decipher what is going on inside our bodies? The only reliable way is to be aware of all the symptoms and be guided by how you feel. Here are some of the highlights:

- Chest pains, palpitations (racing heartbeat)
- Insomnia, disturbed sleep
- Migraine, severe headaches
- Loss of hearing, vertigo, dizziness, tinnitus
- Depression, low mood, anxiety
- Loss of confidence, loss of joy
- Anger, rage, mood swings
- Confusion, brain fog, memory loss
- Vaginal dryness, discharge, bleeding
- Loss of sex drive, painful sex
- UTIs, pelvic inflammation
- Thrush, cystitis, vaginal and clitoral atrophy, vaginal itching
- Dry eyes, blurred vision
- Sore mouth and tongue
- Aching joints, muscle weakness
- Loss of bone density
- Breast pain and tenderness
- Bloating, swelling of the hands and feet
- Dry skin, loss of skin elasticity
- Itchy skin, skin rashes
- Brittle nails, hair loss and thinning

- Abdominal weight gain
- Night sweats
- And . . . hot flushes

Do any of these resonate with you? How many did you check off? Could any health issues – from severe health concerns to smaller niggles – be less about a mainstream, recognised health problem and have more to do with a hidden hormonal imbalance? It's useful to keep a note of symptoms and their severity as a menopausal monitor. Keeping a diary or symptom tracker is an invaluable starting point. The Balance Menopause App (see page 307) is a good resource to help with this and also has a good preappointment checklist if you are planning on having discussions with your doctor.

Make a note of how you feel morning, noon and night. Jot down every niggle – from aching joints to anxiety, mood swings to dry skin, and heart palpitations to tinnitus. Unfortunately, every part of the body can be affected by lowering oestrogen and it's certainly not all about hot flushes! I have never had a hot flush in my life and yet I was very definitely suffering from lowered oestrogen. Far from being 'textbook' as a perimenopausal woman, my symptoms were easily confused with stress. I lived on painkillers, comforted by chocolate and caffeine for many years – and my work life, home life, relationships and marriage suffered. I wish I had known then what I know now.

I've lost count of the number of women who've told me of their long, painful (and costly) journey towards discovering the truth. Women who have undergone expensive electrocardiograms (ECGs) and heart scans, taken beta blockers and been prescribed antidepressants for their heart palpitations and menopausal low mood, when they could have had these so swiftly and effectively fixed by just a bit more oestrogen. I've spoken to many consultant cardiologists who have never considered loss of oestrogen when it comes to assessing a 40-something woman presenting with heart palpitations. Not to mention the psychiatrists and mental health practitioners who don't consider the loss of oestrogen in brain receptors before prescribing mood-numbing antidepressant drugs to middle-aged women. With such widespread and commonly occurring menopausal symptoms, surely a three-month trial of safe, natural, body-identical oestrogen (inexpensive and widely available on the NHS) would be a more obvious first course of action, before upscaling to medications that carry significant, sometimes addictive, side effects and greater cost? Surely this has to be a more sensible, safe and effective first course of action?

Not only are the often lengthy delays in menopausal symptom diagnosis time-consuming, worrying and life-limiting (many women leave jobs and give up careers they love when they find themselves no longer able to cope), but these medical appointments, reviews with specialists and clinical tests are costing our already overloaded health service an absolute fortune in wasted time and money. Let's hope greater awareness among our medical practitioners, together with more patient knowledge and advocacy for women's rights will help more women get the care they need going forward.

If replacing hormones as they decline with age is such an obvious course of action to alleviate the symptoms that occur when we lose them, why has there been such a lack of support for midlife women in this area? It would seem fairly obvious that putting back our own hormones when we need them is both safe and sensible, in much the same way that allowing someone with diabetes to replace their insulin, or those with a thyroid issue to top up their thyroxine, is routine. There are two answers to this:

Firstly, the lack of comprehensive menopause training at medical school for our doctors, which comes back to my earlier observation about the low prioritising of women's healthcare generally (see page 39). In my opinion, it is scandalous that medics spend months learning about pregnancy, antenatal and postnatal care, yet have just a few lectures, at best, learning about menopause care. Not every woman will have a baby, while every woman (should she live long enough) will have a menopause. Half a doctor's patients are women, so very much more knowledge needs to be shared with medics in this area so they can better support their increasingly ageing, female clientele.

The second reason is the perpetuation of the myth that replacing our natural hormones leads to a high risk of breast cancer, which I'll debunk below. As a vocal and unapologetic advocate of HRT, I've found myself drawn into discussions on its safety many times. These conversations are often fraught with the challenges of having to consistently rebut deeply ingrained misinformation and fear. Let me say this out loud:

HRT has consistently been found to be overwhelmingly safe, effective and *beneficial* for the vast majority of women.

Even on the most basic of evidence, it would seem unrealistic that HRT (principally the hormone oestrogen) causes breast cancer. Young women have higher levels of oestrogen than older women, yet rates of breast cancer are higher among older women. Why would this be the case if oestrogen was the cause? Surely it would be the other way around? Could breast cancer be triggered by a *lack* of oestrogen?

Before we dig deep into the benefits of replacing missing hormones, let's first correct some of the more prevalent misinformation when it comes to the menopause with a few factual responses to the most common concerns.

Common HRT Myths

Myth: HRT increases the risk of breast cancer

Truth bomb: incorrect. An important study published in the *Journal of the American Medical Association* (*JAMA*) in 2020 showed that women who take oestrogen-only HRT for more than 20 years have a *lower* risk of developing breast cancer and a *lower* risk of dying from breast cancer, compared to women not taking HRT. There is a small increased risk of developing breast cancer in women who take oestrogen with a synthetic progestogen (the older form of HRT), but *not* with the newer form of micronised (body-identical) progesterone, most commonly prescribed today. Further information on this can be found in the References on page 317.

The study that sparked this dangerous link between HRT and breast cancer was the now widely discredited Women's Health Initiative study published in 2002. The study was released to the press before it had been correctly reviewed, leading to a frenzy of headlines incorrectly making wild and worrying claims connecting HRT to breast cancer, CHD, stroke, dementia and more. So pervasive is the misinformation from this study that I continue to hear it being quoted time and again, often by high-profile doctors, on podcasts or in the media. Not surprisingly, the prescribing of HRT fell off a cliff back in 2002 and many women stopped taking it overnight. Doctors became unfamiliar with prescribing it and are now often wary as a result. Much has been written about this since (I have extensively covered the subject in previous books, including *The Good Menopause Guide* and my e-guides *Healthy Menopause* and *The Truth About HRT*), so I won't repeat myself here; suffice to say that when data from this study was re-evaluated some years later, replacement oestrogen was actually linked to a *lower* risk of breast cancer (as well as many other significant health benefits). By then, though, the 'dangers' of HRT had become ingrained in public perception and the damage to midlife women's healthcare had already been done. Interestingly, although HRT prescribing pretty much stopped overnight when this study was released over 20 years ago, rates of breast cancer have continued to climb since, rising from 1 in 12 women back then to 1 in 7 now. Not something you'd expect to see if HRT were actually the cause, or even a contributing factor.

Truth be told, HRT has not been shown to cause cancer, but it has been shown to prevent it. Here in the UK, one in seven women taking HRT will develop breast cancer – and one in seven women not taking HRT will develop breast cancer. There will always be women who start their HRT only to receive a breast cancer diagnosis shortly afterwards. Given the fact that breast cancer tumours tend to be very slow growing, often taking years from inception to detection, it seems that lifestyle, or perhaps genetic predisposition (or a combination of risk factors), and not HRT are the more likely culprits. Of course, it's easier to blame a new medication than our own, long love affair with alcohol, a poor diet, obesity, tobacco or lack of exercise.

Myth: HRT simply delays the menopause

Truth bomb: incorrect. Replacing hormones during menopause will ease the symptoms of lost oestrogen while it is taken. Once stopped, symptoms will return if they would naturally be experienced (bearing in mind, menopause symptoms can last a decade or more). It's the same as taking a painkiller for a headache – the analgesia works to stop the pain, it doesn't delay the pain. If the painkiller wears off, you might still have the headache if it is a long-lasting one. If the headache has passed, you will feel fine. It's the same with HRT – it does not delay the march of the menopause.

Myth: HRT builds up in the body

Truth bomb: incorrect. HRT only works for as long as you are taking it – much like the synthetic hormones in the contraceptive pill. It does not accumulate in the body and, if you miss a day, you will be similarly 'unprotected'. This is why body-identical HRT patches are so helpful for many women, as they deliver a continuous dose of hormones through the skin, ensuring you never run short until you need to replace the patch.

Myth: HRT causes weight gain

Truth bomb: there is no good evidence to support this, although in the first few weeks of taking HRT some women can experience bloating as their body adjusts to having its hormones back. This doesn't happen for all women and usually settles quickly, sometimes with a slight adjustment to the type or dose of HRT being taken. In terms of weight management, women on HRT often lose weight as they have more motivation and energy, and less joint pain, so are able to be more active. In the infamous Women's Health Initiative study, one of the correct findings was that women actually lost weight when taking HRT compared to those taking the placebo (dummy pill). Oestrogen also helps with a healthier fat distribution, so the body stores less abdominal fat (the dangerous kind linked to a higher risk of heart disease, type 2 diabetes and stroke). Many women find they get their waistline back once taking HRT and it can also help reduce 'muffin top'.

Myth: you can't take HRT due to deep vein thrombosis (DVT) or migraine
Truth bomb: incorrect. This used to be the case before the introduction of modern, transdermal HRT delivery methods, allowing hormones to be absorbed through the skin from a patch, gel or spray. The older tablet form of HRT is associated with a slight increased risk of blood clotting, which is why it is contraindicated for anyone with a history of DVT, stroke or migraine. However, transdermal HRT is delivered directly into the bloodstream and does not go via the liver, where clotting factors are produced, so there is no risk of clot. Anyone who is denied HRT for these reasons should see another GP or healthcare professional who understands how blood clots are formed in the liver and is informed on the way transdermal delivery systems work in medicine.

Myth: I can't take HRT as I have had breast cancer
Truth bomb: incorrect. If you have had breast cancer some specialists will still prescribe certain forms of HRT. Women with breast cancer (past or present) can use localised vaginal hormones,

which are different from systemic HRT (the kind that circulates around the body), as they stay within the vagina to help ease symptoms of dryness, irritation and recurrent bladder and pelvic infections. Care for breast cancer patients and for those following treatment needs a careful, specialist and individualised approach from medics experienced in this area. It is perfectly possible to take HRT following a breast cancer diagnosis and treatment. I have listed a few helpful resources on page 308. These women's health specialists will often also help women who have other specific issues previously considered no-go areas, such as endometriosis.

Myth: I can't take HRT over the age of 60

Truth bomb: incorrect. It used to be that the NICE guidelines on menopause advised 'the lowest dose of HRT for the shortest length of time'. These were revised in 2015, although some doctors seem not to be aware of this. According to the NICE guidelines published in 2015 (the latest update at the time of writing), HRT can continue to be prescribed for as long as the benefits outweigh the risks. There is no upper age limit and there is no set end date. Some GPs may be reluctant to prescribe HRT for the first time over the age of 60, as there is likely to have been a gap of many years without hormones, so any replacements would need to be given in smaller amounts and carefully monitored to allow the body to readjust. My own mother actually went back on to HRT at the age of 80, having been taken off it during her sixties because 'you don't need this anymore'. She now sleeps well and feels much better for it.

In 2017, the North American Menopause Society issued guidelines stating that, 'Hormone therapy does not need to be routinely discontinued in women older than 60 or 65 years and can be considered beyond 65 years for persistent vasomotor symptoms, quality of life issues, or prevention of osteoporosis after appropriate evaluation and counselling the benefits and risks . . .'. The view of both the International and British Menopause Societies is much the same.

Myth: I should delay taking HRT for as long as possible

Truth bomb: incorrect. Studies show that the earlier HRT is started, the greater the protective health benefits. Research published in the journal *Alzheimer's Research and Therapy* in 2020 looked at data from over a thousand women as part of the European Prevention of Alzheimer's Dementia initiative, which showed that HRT is associated with better memory, cognition and larger brain volumes in later life – and that this was most effective when women started taking it during perimenopause. See page 93 for more about the protective role of HRT.

Myth: compounded, bio-identical hormones are safer

Truth bomb: incorrect. The craze for highly-priced, so-called 'bio-identical' hormones has been driven by the fear of synthetic hormones carrying a slightly greater risk of cancer and blood clots, probably due to their synthetic progestin component. However, modern transdermal oestrogen and micronised progesterone are body-identical (they are also sometimes confusingly referred to as bio-identical) and are exactly the same as those found naturally circulating around a woman's body.

The 'menopause shelf' in the supplement world is a crowded space; there is much money to be made from this new-found segment of the population hungry for help – and the profit motive is a strong commercial driver. Financial incentive can influence everything from organisations that accept commercial sponsorship to private medics who seem keener to cash in by selling unregulated hormones than direct women to the NHS, where they should be treated cheaply and well. I do not advocate buying expensive unregulated and untrialled 'bio-identical' hormones made in a compounding chemist as it is unclear what is in these preparations or how safe they are. For safety, I would only ever use a regulated form of HRT that has undergone extensive testing. This is especially important when it comes to progesterone, needed to protect the lining of the womb against uterine cancer. Progesterone creams that you rub onto the skin should be avoided for this reason, as there is no clinical data to show sufficient is absorbed through the skin to give adequate protection against developing cancer.

Myth: HRT is not natural

Truth bomb: hmmm. I hear this one a lot, especially from those trying to sell me herbal menopause 'solutions'. I completely agree that some herbal remedies, such as sage, agnus castus, red clover, dong quai and black cohosh can help some women with some specific symptoms, such as hot flushes (and I'll explore these on page 97), but I am a human being, not a plant, so a more natural and body-compatible approach would be to replace my own hormones with body-identical hormones; albeit plant-derived, they are the same as those produced by the body, not entirely different herbs. There is scant large-scale evidence for the efficacy of herbal menopause remedies (beyond what you would expect from a placebo), but that's not to say they won't help relieve symptoms. What no herb or vitamin supplement can do, of course, is actually replace oestrogen. Only oestrogen itself can do that. If you do choose a herbal supplement, look for those that carry the Traditional Herbal Registration (THR) symbol – the leading certification scheme for herbal products in the UK – to ensure it's regulated for safety.

Myth: HRT is only for hot flushes

Truth bomb: incorrect. Gosh, how long have you got here?! As we saw on page 77, the list of symptoms experienced by women with lowering rates of hormones is almost endless. HRT will reduce *all* symptoms associated with lowering levels of hormones – not just hot flushes – simply by adding these hormones back into the body.

Myth: HRT is just for menopause symptoms

Truth bomb: incorrect. Although, technically, HRT is usually only prescribed for the relief of menopausal symptoms (such as those listed on page 77), it also confers other health benefits – many of which are very significant. For example, women on HRT have a 50 per cent reduced risk of CHD and stroke (that one statistic alone should be enough to make the entire medical world sit up and pay attention, as CHD is the biggest killer of women – far more so than breast cancer). HRT also helps with osteoporosis, an extremely painful and life-limiting bone disease, as oestrogen is uniquely needed to retain elasticity within the bones, which helps us 'bounce' and not fracture when we fall; an important fact often overlooked when discussing osteoporosis treatment and care. Some of the most exciting studies have been in the area of brain health, cognitive decline, dementia and Alzheimer's disease. The research here, including that around testosterone, is very promising.

When it comes to cancer, oestrogen-only HRT has been shown to be breast-cancer-protective, as well as reducing the risk of colon cancer by around one third. A 30-year study of 300,000 women in the UK, aged 46–65 years found that women taking oestrogen-only and combined HRT had, on average, a 9 per cent lower risk of death from any cause. Women on HRT not only have a significantly lower death rate from breast cancer than those not taking it, they also live longer overall. Instead of talking about the risks of taking HRT, perhaps we should start talking more about the risk of *not* taking HRT.

Myth: testosterone is a male hormone

Truth bomb: incorrect. Women make *three times* more testosterone in their ovaries than oestrogen, and testosterone receptors are literally everywhere in a woman's body. Often only cited for sex drive, we also need testosterone for our eye health, brain function (especially word recall and memory), improved mood, heart health, muscle mass, bone density and glucose metabolism. When it comes to testosterone prescribing, it is truly scandalous that so many women are being denied access to having their own natural hormone back in later life.

HRT: What to Expect

When we talk about female hormones in general, and HRT in particular, we're usually talking about two, or possibly three, different ones: oestrogen, progesterone and testosterone. Each of these is fundamentally important for women at every stage of life, whether we produce them naturally when younger or replace them with body-identical versions as we age. Since I first started writing about hormone health and the menopause many years ago, lots of good resources have become available exploring these hormones and how they support our health, so I won't go into detail here. However, if you'd like to learn more, there is lots of information on my website: lizearlewellbeing.com/bshlinks. I've also detailed some of the trusted experts I turn to for up-to-date, evidence-based information on HRT on page 308 and won't dwell too much on the prescribing of HRT here. However, I should say that for anyone dipping a toe into the world of replacement hormones, it's not always an easy journey. HRT is not a 'one-size-fits-all' treatment. You may be one of the lucky ones (like me) who finds immediate symptom relief or gets a good night's sleep from rubbing on your first bit of oestrogen gel, or it may take months of trial and error, adjusting the type and dose of your hormones. It's common to start with oestrogen (and progesterone if you have a uterus), usually in the most modern, safest, transdermal (through the skin) form. This could be a gel, a spray or a patch – they all contain the same yam-based, body-identical oestrogen.

All HRT dosages, regimens and durations need to be prescribed individually, with an annual review where you can discuss symptoms, changes, updates and so on. We're all different and have varying levels of hormones and ways of absorbing them. What works for me might not work for you, and vice versa. Once the dose is right though, menopausal symptoms can be fully relieved and the future risks of heart disease, osteoporosis, clinical depression and type 2 diabetes are all lowered.

So how do you know what is the right dose for you? The obvious answer is, it's whatever dose effectively relieves your symptoms so that you feel completely well again. Oestradiol level blood tests can give a snapshot of what is happening in your blood at any moment in time, but are not especially accurate if you take oestrogen as a tablet, as oestrogen is metabolised into different types when it is digested. However, these tests can be helpful for transdermal oestrogen to see if it's being absorbed properly and getting into the bloodstream. Generally, levels need to be over 250pmol/L and a few women need to have a level above 1,000pmol/L. Keep in mind that oestrogen levels can surge during perimenopause as well as during your period. In comparison, levels of oestrogen naturally skyrocket to around 65,000pmol/L during pregnancy, so menopausal levels are very much lower than this. Studies show that younger women going through perimeno-pause often need higher levels of oestradiol than older women, so you may need to discuss this more thoroughly with your (hope-fully well-informed) doctor.

Some women might also need higher doses than others as oestrogen is absorbed differently through the skin; some absorb patches better than gels, for example. Different brands can also vary in absorption, even if they contain exactly the same ingredi-ents. It can be a minefield! To achieve a specific oestradiol level, some of us may only need a very low dose; others a much higher one. All transdermal HRT is absorbed via a network of tiny capil-laries which supply blood and nutrients to the skin. The depth and numbers of these capillaries is different in all of us. Other factors affect absorption too, such as skin thickness, how hydrated the skin is and even body temperature. Skin is designed to be a barrier and keep things out of the body, and some of us have skin that's more effective at doing this than others, meaning our trans-dermal absorption rate will be different. Ethnicity also affects skin absorption, with one study finding that those from a Hispanic background had the best absorption rate, followed by Caucasians, Asians and finally those from an Afro-Caribbean background. It's important to be aware of this as you may find you need more than the recommended amount to help your symptoms.

Your dose of progesterone does not usually require as much tweaking or adjustment and there's no strong evidence to suggest that those on a higher dose of oestrogen need a higher dose of progesterone to complement it. The rate of absorption into the bloodstream often means that a higher dose of oestrogen given ends up as an average dose once it's actually been absorbed. Some women will experience bleeding when replacing progesterone, regardless of their oestrogen dose. Persistent bleeding could be a sign of something that needs investigation, but bear in mind that bleeding is common during the first three to six months of starting or changing the dose of HRT, and is not usually a sign of anything untoward. If you have a womb, you will always need progesterone alongside. Many patches combine both oestrogen and the synthetic form of progesterone, and can be a handy dual option.

Testosterone (when it's prescribed) is usually given once a woman is happily settled into her oestrogen/progesterone regime. The starting dose tends to be 5mg of cream or gel daily, rubbed into the thigh at bedtime. A blood test is then usual after three to six months to check the level of testosterone and sex hormone binding globulin (SHBG) to determine your free androgen index (FAI). If levels are low, your dose may be increased. Side effects are rare if levels of testosterone and FAI remain in the female range.

Vaginal HRT is also hugely helpful for treating and preventing genitourinary syndrome of menopause (GSM), a newer term recognising symptoms such as dryness, burning, irritation, pain, urinary urge and incontinence. It is easily and safely remedied with either vaginal oestrogen in the form of creams, rings or pessaries (such as Vagifem), or Intrarosa, a plant-derived vaginal pessary containing DHEA, a 'precursor' hormone, meaning the body converts it to testosterone and oestrogen. Absorbed locally, Intrarosa improves GSM as well as lifting libido and making sex more physically comfortable.

> **The health risks of replacing our own naturally occurring hormones are extremely small. The health benefits that can be gained are extremely large.**

Should All Women Take HRT?

That is the million-dollar question! I certainly believe that all midlife women should be offered the choice and share in the decision-making here. Research is being published all the time that shows the protective role of HRT and that the sooner it is started, the better the outcome for our overall health and a reduced risk of death from all causes. Here are just a few facts and figures that support this:

Heart disease: HRT cuts the risk of women's biggest killer by 50 per cent – far and away more effective than something like statins, commonly accepted as being beneficial despite providing far less benefit and more side effects.

Osteoporosis: one of the biggest killers of women, painful and debilitating, it's a very serious midlife health concern. Oestrogen plays a fundamentally important role here for bone tensile strength and elasticity, meaning bones are less likely to snap or fracture. Unlike the more commonly prescribed bisphosphonates, which have a history of being effective for five years or so before actually *increasing* the risk of atypical femoral fractures, oestrogen improves our bodies' bone resistance to fractures forever. This needs to be much more widely known and urgently discussed to benefit our bones.

Type 2 diabetes: another major killer (not to mention cause of blindness and limb amputation). Oestrogen helps control insulin sensitivity and blood glucose levels, decreasing the incidence of type 2 diabetes.

Cancer: the use of HRT is associated with a 33 per cent reduction in the risk of colorectal cancer, also known as bowel cancer, and research published in the *Journal of Clinical Medicine Research* in 2022 shows replacement oestrogen to be associated with 'a significantly reduced risk' of developing breast cancer too.

UTIs: recurrent UTIs are common as we age, often due to the changing pH around the bladder and urethra thinning internal tissues and increasing inflammation. Localised oestrogen inserted into the vagina is an extremely safe and effective way to prevent and treat not only UTIs, but also vaginal dryness and atrophy (where there's a drying, shrivelling and hardening of the vaginal tissues).

Alzheimer's disease: some of the most exciting new research is centring on brain function and the ability of oestrogen to stave off dementia and cognitive decline. Research from the University of Arizona Center for Innovation in Brain Science found that women on HRT had a staggering 58 per cent lower risk of Alzheimer's, with the greatest benefits seen in those who had taken HRT for at least six years, with a 79 per cent reduced risk of developing Alzheimer's and a 77 per cent risk reduction for Parkinson's.

To my mind, replacing declining hormones in some shape or form is fundamental for both our current midlife health and for later-life disease prevention. Many medics are now even looking at the preventative use of oestrogen, for example, which may be able to head off symptoms earlier in life before they even have an impact. Should this also be considered by women who say they're sailing through the menopause without a single symptom (although I have yet to meet an older woman who does not have at least *one* of the many health issues on my previous, very long, list of low-oestrogen symptoms)? This is all up for future discussion as we don't yet have the data, but I do suspect that the conversations my daughters will be having with their GPs in years to come will be very different from those of my generation.

I do know that some women, even those suffering with symptoms, simply may not want to replace their hormones, or perhaps are undergoing some form of medical treatment that contraindicates it. Those who decide against HRT may be offered a low-dose antidepressant, as these can reduce some cases of hot flushes and night sweats; however, they can further reduce libido and leave a feeling of 'numbness'. Women with menopausal symptoms should not be offered antidepressants as their first line of treatment, as there is no conclusive evidence that they benefit menopause-related symptoms. Other prescription medications might include gabapentin, pregabalin and metformin, which can all be of some benefit, but do come with side effects.

Alternatives to HRT: What Really Works?

As someone who champions natural remedies and a drug-free life-style as far as possible, I'm often asked whether HRT is the only way to help with perimenopause and menopausal symptoms. The short answer is yes. To put it bluntly, only by replacing hormones can we replace our hormones.

However, for those wishing to avoid HRT or medication, for whatever reason, there are some natural supplements that can help. These won't replace oestrogen, but they may help take the edge off some of the health issues caused by having an insufficiency.

Herbs that can help in midlife

Some herbs and supplements contain phytoestrogens, derived from plants ('phyto' coming from the Greek work 'phyton', mean-ing plant). These include black cohosh, red clover and soya isofla-vones. It's unclear how these work in the body and there's really not enough clinical evidence to confirm whether they're effective. They may work for some women – or they may not. Often the results are no more impressive than taking a placebo. These kinds of supplements are also unregulated, so it's not always possible to know precisely what a product contains – or how effective it will be. Always buy from a well-established, trusted brand that prides itself on independent research, product quality and safety testing. Be wise when choosing what to take – don't waste money buying supplements from dubious online sources or private clinics spouting spurious claims with zero clinical evidence. Your health is far too important for that.

These are some of the herbs reputed to be helpful for easing some menopause symptoms for some women. Although some of these may improve some symptoms, they will not improve future health and reduce risk of future diseases in the way that HRT is proven to do.

Chaste tree (*Vitex Agnes castus*): said to help with mood swings, tension and anxiety. Shown to have potential benefit for reducing breast pain and easing premenstrual syndrome, possibly by decreasing levels of the hormone prolactin, which helps rebalance other hormones (including oestrogen and progesterone). However, studies have been small and not randomised controlled.

Black cohosh (*Cimicifuga racemose*): may help reduce mood swings, irritability, vaginal dryness, palpitations and night sweats, as well as help with premenstrual migraine (which can become more severe during menopause). However, a review of 16 randomised controlled trials, totalling over 2,000 perimenopausal or postmenopausal women showed no significant difference between black cohosh and placebo in the frequency of hot flushes, although the authors did suggest the effect on other symptoms such as night sweats and bone health should be further investigated. High doses have been associated with liver failure.

Dong quai (*Angelica sinensis*): used in traditional Chinese medicine (TCM) and recommended by some herbalists to ease insomnia and sleep disturbed by hot flushes and night sweats. Nicknamed the 'female ginseng', dong quai contains trans-ferulic acid which may have anti-inflammatory effects and decrease blood clotting.

Red clover (*Trifolium pratense*): has been shown to help improve some symptoms in some studies, but there is insufficient conclusive evidence. A potent antioxidant also being studied for potential anti-cancer properties, red clover isoflavone extracts are often touted as beneficial for bones and cardiovascular health, but no robust studies support this.

Sage (*Salvia officinalis*): one of the most popular menopausal herbs used to help reduce excessive sweating, hot flushes and night sweats. Small studies have shown benefit for hot flushes, possibly due to its oestrogenic flavonoids. Sage contains thujone, a chemical that can cause seizures and liver damage, so is possibly unsafe taken in high doses or for a long time. Sage can also interact with other medications, so always discuss, with your doctor before supplementing.

Soya isoflavones: extracted from soya beans, a natural source of phytoestrogens (plant oestrogens). A small, observational study published in the *Journal of Mid-Life Health* in 2022 concluded that soya isoflavone supplementation improved some menopause symptoms by around 40 per cent, with most benefit being seen in perimenopausal women. Some say the best form of supplements are where the soya has been fermented, similar to many of the soya foods eaten by women in Eastern countries, where rates of menopausal symptoms appear to be lower than in the West, such as natto, miso, tempeh and tofu. However, a Cochrane review from 2013 found no firm evidence that eating soya foods eased hot flushes, but did suggest that supplements containing genistein, one of the main isoflavones in soya, was worth further investigation.

Other herbs often cited as being helpful include fenugreek (*Trigonella foenum-graecum*), hops (*Humulus lupulus*), lemon balm (*Melissa officinalis*), valerian (*Valeriana officinalis*) and evening primrose oil (*Oenothera biennis*).

Overall, the clinical evidence for these herbs is not strong, but that's not to say that some women don't find them helpful, maybe even more than you'd expect from a placebo. If buying, choose a respected brand and look for the THR logo on the pack (see earlier mention on page 88).

Nutrition for Menopause

Times of hormonal change, pregnancy, perimenopause, menopause and beyond are all times of life that call on greater nutritional resources to support the body. These times are definitely not for calorie restriction or dieting. Instead, focus on eating more of the healthy fats, as these provide important levels of essential fatty acids and cholesterol, the building blocks of our hormones. Without healthy fats, we can't create the hormones we need to age well. So, ditch anything labelled 'low-fat' or, even worse, 'fat-free' and focus instead on unprocessed fats from healthy, natural foods, such as eggs (especially nutrient-dense egg yolks), full-fat yoghurt, sheep and goats' cheeses, oily fish, pastured poultry and red meat – especially wild game and organ meats (such as offal).

What we eat (and drink) plays a large part in menopause management, with an emphasis on more protein and plant fibre, with low or no sugar being central to this. Eating foods with a low glycaemic index (GI), such as brown rice instead of white rice, helps reduce sugar spikes and supports the pancreas by keeping insulin levels steady. However, brown rice does contain 1.5 times more arsenic than white rice. As we'll explore in Chapter 7, good gut health is also vitally important and the microbiome is also involved in the menopause.

I'll focus more on food and supplements in the next few chapters, but here's the top-line on a few nutrients we should be prioritising when it comes to menopause and symptoms caused by oestrogen decline:

B-complex

Essential for regulating the central nervous system, controlling anxiety and giving us energy, the B vitamins are often referred to as the 'B-complex' as they work synergistically with each other and are often best taken together. They include:

- B1: thiamine
- B2: riboflavin
- B3: niacin
- B5: pantothenic acid
- B6: pyridoxine
- B7: biotin
- B9: folate and folic acid
- B12: cobalamin

All are widely found in whole foods (with the exception of B12, only naturally found in animal produce and yeast) and all are depleted by food processing.

Calcium

This is widely available in many foods (notably yoghurt, milk and ricotta cheese), so few of us are likely to be calcium-deficient if we eat plenty of these, although supplies do dwindle in later life as we don't process it so well as we age. Although dairy products are the highest and most traditional sources, calcium is also found in tofu, oranges, cabbage, broccoli and other brassicas, lettuce leaves, such as rocket and watercress, almonds and tahini (sesame seed paste). If using synthetically fortified plant-based alternatives to dairy, do make sure they are enriched with added calcium.

As our bodies can't make calcium, we must obtain it from our diets and it diminishes with age. Calcium is essential for making strong bones and helping to guard against osteoporosis. Repeated studies show that low levels are linked to low bone mass and high fracture rates. Although we might not be aware of the importance of this while young, our ability to store calcium in our bones switches off in our mid- to late twenties, meaning we can't 'load' calcium into our bones in later life. All we can hope to do, at best, is prevent calcium loss by making sure we eat sufficient amounts. This is why it's so important our daughters and younger members of the family and friends know the dangers of a restricted diet (especially if dairy-free) during their teenage years and their early twenties.

Menopause also saps our calcium supplies, meaning we need to be eating more – so be sure to eat plenty of calcium-rich foods on a daily basis. If taking supplements, space these out during the day as calcium is better absorbed in small doses. Calcium also needs vitamin D in order to be converted into the hormone calcitriol (also known as the 'active' form of vitamin D), either from sunlight or from animal foods or supplements, and many food supplements combine the two nutrients together.

Vitamin D

Also referred to as 'calciferol', vitamin D is also known as a fat-soluble vitamin but is actually a hormone (a prohormone, to be precise) with many varied and critical roles in the body. It helps calcium absorption in the gut and protects against osteoporosis by enabling strong bone remineralisation, as well as maintaining muscle strength. It is also fundamentally important for our immune systems, as evidenced during the Covid-19 pandemic when those with the lowest levels of vitamin D were found to be among the most severely affected. Long-term deficiency is also thought to play a role in the development of autoimmune issues (including rheumatoid arthritis), diabetes and asthma. As it is a fat-soluble nutrient, it is affected by any gastrointestinal conditions, such as irritable bowel syndrome (IBS), which affect our ability to absorb fats. Others at risk of deficiency include the elderly (our ability to process vitamin D decreases with age, especially among women over the age of 60) and those with a higher level of body fat. Being above a healthy weight dramatically increases our need for vitamin D, as does having a genetic variance (SNP or 'snip' – see page 49) that lowers the way we absorb vitamin D.

We can find the two main forms of vitamin D from foods, supplements and sunshine. Vitamin D2 comes from plant sources (such as mushrooms exposed to sunlight, and algae), while vitamin D3 is found in animal foods (notably oily fish and cod liver oil).

Studies show the D3 form to be better at raising vitamin D levels in the blood. Sunlight also creates D3 through skin synthesis, although it's hard to be precise about how much we need to absorb to give us adequate vitamin D protection. The current consensus seems to be 5–30 minutes of middle-of-the-day sun exposure, either daily or at least twice a week to the face, arms, hands and legs, without sunscreen. Pigmentation also reduces our ability to absorb vitamin D, so those with darker skin need to spend more time in the sun for their vitamin D supplies than those who are naturally pale. This is obviously at odds with current thinking of the skin cancer lobby and those concerned with premature skin ageing, so the potentially safer bet is to eat vitamin D-rich foods and/or take a food supplement alongside some sun exposure (but never burning the skin). Vitamin D3 supplements are often combined with vitamin K2, which not only assists blood clotting and muscle function, but also ensures calcium is absorbed more effectively to reach the bone mass, while also preventing arterial calcification – helping to keep both heart and bones healthier.

Iodine

This is essential for making thyroid hormones, which keep cells healthy as well as regulating our metabolism. Levels in foods vary depending on where they came from. For example, intensive farming has depleted iodine in most soils, so plant uptake is much less than it was a few decades ago. Good sources include seaweed, white fish (such as haddock and cod), shellfish, 'iodised' salt, dairy produce including milk and yoghurt, and eggs. Algae supplements are a useful source of iodine for all midlifers. Low levels of iodine in the diet can lead to an underactive thyroid (hypothyroidism), causing tiredness, weight gain, sensitivity to cold, brain fog and poor memory (often confused with menopausal symptoms). Research shows that iodine can help weight loss and blood-sugar management by its ability to slow the breakdown of carbohydrates. Wakame is the type of seaweed that contains the most fucoxanthin, the fat-fighting bioactive shown to increase metabolism.

Iron

Important for energy and muscle strength, iron fortifies red blood cells and, without it, we can't produce enough haemoglobin – the substance that carries oxygen around the body to help sustain us. Too little iron in the system means that we end up feeling weak, tired and irritable (even more so if we are lacking oestrogen!). There are two forms of dietary iron: heme and non-heme. Heme iron comes from haemoglobin and so is found in meat and seafood (the redder the meat, the more heme iron it contains, such as beef steak, chicken leg or liver). Non-heme iron is from plant sources such as kidney beans, dried apricots and wheatgerm. It is not as well absorbed by the body as heme iron, so plant-based eaters risk a deficiency. Calcium also interferes with iron absorption, whereas vitamin C improves it, so drinking a small glass of orange juice while eating steak would be a better choice than a glass of milk.

Magnesium

This mighty mineral is involved with over 300 critical biochemical processes in the body and is a fundamentally important nutrient for us all, yet is decreased (along with oestrogen) during the menopause and beyond, making associated symptoms more noticeable. Magnesium influences mood, supports healthy bones by boosting bone matrix calcification (increased bone strength) and regulates hormones. Magnesium also plays a role in promoting better sleep by regulating our circadian rhythms (more on sleep in Chapter 10) and increasing muscle relaxation. Good magnesium levels (alongside zinc and selenium) have also been shown to help alleviate depression, lift mood and ease anxiety. Foods with the highest levels include dark chocolate, avocados, almonds, cashews, Brazil nuts, lentils, chickpeas, soya beans, natto and tofu.

Omega-3s

The omega-3 fats docosahexaenoic acid (DHA) and eicosapentaenoic acid (EPA) have been shown to protect against cognitive decline in older age, as well as help reduce the frequency of menopausal hot flushes and depression. High-quality fish oil supplements are a less expensive alternative to eating fish and provide a measured amount of these important fats. Typically, look for supplements containing roughly twice as much EPA as DHA (vegans can look for algae-based supplements, which although not as well absorbed, do give some helpful nutritional brain benefit).

Lifestyle Hacks to Live Well

Of course, managing our health during midlife and far beyond doesn't just include an investigation into hormones (or vitamins and herbs). There's more to it than that when it comes to managing menopausal symptoms, as well as midlife ways to live well. Some of the therapies shown to be most useful for supporting women during the menopause include yoga and Qigong (which I'll cover in more detail in Chapter 9), mindfulness and meditation (which I'll feature more of in Chapter 8), as well as behavioural therapies such as cognitive behavioural therapy (CBT), which has been shown, for some, to reduce the frequency and duration of hot flushes triggered by stress or poor sleep. Acupuncture has also been shown to be helpful for some menopausal symptoms, and many midlifers (myself included) are fans of the restorative powers of reflexology, sound baths and shiatsu massage.

It's also no secret that I'm a fan of cold-water therapy and can often be seen on my Instagram dipping in the freshwater pond at the end of my garden, having a cold shower, taking a sea swim when by the coast or even booking in for a crazily cold -130°C cryotherapy session – all highly effective ways to boost endorphins and the 'happy hormone' serotonin in the brain, resulting in a post-shock 'high' and a genuine glow. While there's not much data on relief for menopause symptoms specifically, cold exposure brings with it many benefits for midlifers (far beyond combatting hot flushes). Dipping in cold water (even a 60-second cold shower) benefits blood circulation and the lymphatic system, helping to improve the elasticity and responsiveness of veins that can stiffen due to lack of oestrogen. Cold-water dipping also supports the immune system by reducing inflammation and may help guard against dementia by increasing a protein that protects against brain cell death. A further benefit, especially for those living beside the sea, a wild swimming lake or city lido, is that there is often a group of 'wild-swimmers' who gather in the mornings to share the experience, encouraging and supporting those of all ages, but often midlife and beyond. This is also a valuable part of wellbeing – a safe and supportive cold-water community where ideas and experiences are shared, talked through, laughed and cried over, which can be especially helpful around the time of the menopause. See Resources, page 306 for details on where to find a group near you.

Other simple lifestyle habits can also help ease this time of change, including making sleep much more of a priority. Our sleep patterns often change as our hormones fluctuate and we're more likely to wake in the night due to heart palpitations, changes in body temperature (both vasomotor symptoms, otherwise known as hot flushes) or needing to get up for a wee (due to a loss of oestrogen causing a weakness in the bladder cells). This makes prioritising a good night's sleep even more important, and I discuss exactly how to do this in Chapter 10.

For all of you experiencing symptoms driven by hormonal change, I can hand-on-heart say that many of these simple strategies, as well as my all-important HRT, have literally saved my midlife wellbeing, which is why I write so passionately about them here. I wish the same life-changing benefits for you.

Healthy hacks

- Be aware that your hormones will be fluctuating and lowering from your early to mid-forties onwards (sometimes even earlier). Don't be fobbed off with antidepressants for a persistently low mood and always ask your GP if your symptoms could be related to a loss of oestrogen.
- Think of HRT more in terms of health benefits than health risks. The noise around the (largely debunked) links to breast cancer has drowned out the very real health-protective benefits of reduced CHD, osteoporosis, type 2 diabetes, dementia, colon cancer and many other major killers.
- Try a cold shower! It doesn't even have to be for very long. Just dialling down the temperature at the end of your regular shower for a 30–60-second icy blast from top to toe is enough to help hormones lift your mood.

CHAPTER 4

Eating to Age Well

Unlike the millions of self-help and diet books out there, I won't be advocating a specific 'diet plan' or rigid rules in this chapter. What you eat and how your body responds to food is such a personal issue, determined by genetics, individual microbiome, cultural background and personal preferences. Instead, I believe we should be adding more of the good stuff back into our diets, not stripping foods away. So this chapter will focus on the upside of many of my favourite foods for midlife – and why I love them so much. Some of these may surprise you . . .

It's extraordinary that since the release of our globally accepted nutritional 'guidelines' we have become overwhelmingly fatter and fatter. If any company performed as badly over the decades, it would have gone bust a long time ago. The majority of us are over-weight, many very unhealthily so. We've accepted 'plus size' as if it's a normal part of everyday human physiology and anyone daring to point out the risks and very real detriment to health, vitality and lifespan (not to mention the extraordinary burden obesity puts on our already overstretched health services), risks being accused of 'fat shaming'. In reality, the goal must surely be greater health and wellness for all in order to live a longer life.

So what on earth has happened to our modern-day diets? The advent of food processing, the promotion of sugary foods and drinks, the demonising of healthy fats and protein over pro-inflammatory seed oils, the introduction of processed low-fat foods and ultra-processed foods (UPFs – think processed meats, biscuits, crisps, fizzy drinks, mass-produced bread, takeaways or anything premade that comes out of a packet) and their many additives . . . to name just a few of the guilty culprits.

Fats: Friend or Foe?

In the pursuit of getting the right balance between the foods we need more of versus those we need less of, there are a few fundamental food principles I've come to live by over the years that have made the most massive difference to my mood, physical health – and weight. The first is to eat more fat. Yes, really! The fundamental key here is the type of fat. Our bodies need healthy, unprocessed fats, the kind found naturally occurring in everyday foods – not processed, artificially hardened or 'hydrogenated' fats. Once a healthy fat has been hardened or artificially processed, it gets damaged and, in turn, damages us.

As I mentioned earlier, the first book I ever wrote over 30 years ago was *Vital Oils*, which championed the addition of healthy fats in our diets. I am even more evangelical on the subject now than I was back then, having since discovered how data was deliberately skewed to set up fat as our foe, as opposed to sugars.

The high-fat scandal

So why do we fear naturally occurring saturated fat so much? Maybe because it's obvious that the sludgy, gooey stuff in something like a sirloin steak is clearly going to build up the fat layers in our arteries, right? Wrong. One of the greatest travesties of food doctrine followed the publication of an infamous 'fat graph' published in 1948 by Ancel Keys, an American psychologist and statistician, based on a long-term observational study known as The Seven Countries Study. After studying population data on what people ate around the world, Keys proposed that saturated fat was the cause of heart disease. He based his findings on a graph that appeared to show that men who ate the most saturated fat suffered the greatest incidence of heart disease. In fact, Keys cherry-picked his data and ignored the countries that showed high levels of saturated fat intake and lowered heart disease (as well as lower all-cause mortality). Ancel Keys was a powerful champion of this theory, strongly opposed at the time by Professor John Yudkin and others, because the data also showed an equally strong correlation with sugar consumption. Keys won the argument (it's since become known he was paid by the sugar industry at the time), but only because not all of his data was fairly represented. The data could (and should) equally have shown that sugar was the culprit. Professor Yudkin went on to publish a famous book, called *Pure, White and Deadly*, in 1972, stating 'it is the over-consumption of sugar that leads to higher rates of coronary thrombosis, obesity and even some cancers'. His last chapter ends with the line, 'I hope that when you have read this book I shall have convinced you that sugar is really dangerous'. This was a bold and extremely unwelcome statement to the powerful sugar industry and processed-food manufacturers, already making a vast array of highly profitable low-fat, high-sugar foods. Yudkin's efforts to redress the balance and challenge the status quo largely failed and the notion that a high-fat diet is dangerous was seized on and manipulated by the food industry. And so it became firmly enshrined in our global healthcare messaging, aided and abetted by powerful industry lobbyists, targeting everyone from government policymakers to academic research funding and even heart health charities and support groups. Since then, the 'fat graph' of Ancel Keys has been used to demonise saturated fats, when it could just as easily have turned the spotlight on sugar.

When you think about it historically, it seems inconceivable that the natural fats that have nourished us through hundreds, if not thousands, of years – naturally sustaining foods such as olive and coconut oils, butter, lard, ghee, beef dripping and all the rest – could suddenly turn against us. Why would these suddenly become deleterious to our health in favour of highly processed, artificially manufactured, industrially produced seed oils? Did our ancestors die in huge numbers due to heart disease and obesity? No, they did not. Of course, they were susceptible to accidents, injury and dying from basic infections before the advent of life-saving antibiotics, but clogged arteries didn't kill them. In the words of the late Dr Thomas Cleave, surgeon captain and early advocate for healthy fats, 'for a modern disease to be related to an old fashioned food is one of the most ludicrous things I have ever heard in my life'.

What about saturated fat?

In 2010, a major review of 21 scientific studies determined that 'there is no significant evidence for concluding that saturated fats cause heart disease'. In 2014, a study funded by the British Heart

Foundation examined 72 academic studies and found that satu-rated fats were *not* associated with coronary disease risk – which is curious as their website still states (at the time of writing) that 'Too much bad (saturated) fat in your diet can increase your risk of developing heart and circulatory diseases'. The NHS website also still says the same. Hmmm. However, evidence in favour of eating *more* saturated fat continues to roll in, including one study from Holland that followed 35,000 people over a 12-year period and found that the more saturated fat you eat, the lower your risk of dying from cardiovascular disease. In fact, it showed a 13 per cent reduction in death for every 5 per cent increase in energy obtained from saturated fat consumption.

Hydrogenated fats

The work by Ancel Keys and other opponents demonised natural fats, so the food industry seized the chance to turn instead to the (cheaper) polyunsaturated seed oils, such as corn, soya, safflower, sunflower and rapeseed (canola) – more on these below. Their problem though, was that these are all liquid at room temperature, so they're unstable and tricky to work into processed foods. The manufacturing solution was to harden these oils by a process called hydrogenation, which involves heating an oil and combin-ing it with hydrogen atoms. In the food industry, this is known as 'partial hydrogenation' and it also makes the oils last longer, hand-ily improving shelf life. Partially hydrogenated vegetable oils are the backbone of most processed foods on the shelves today – take a stroll through any supermarket and you'll find them in every-thing from the more obvious margarines to fish fingers, biscuits, crisps and pretty much anything in the ready-meal category. It wasn't just the food industry that ditched saturated fats;

consumers were discouraged from using them at home too. Vegetable oils were advocated over butter or lard for frying and even the local chip shop gave up its tasty, highly stable beef dripping in favour of cheaper seed oils. The fact that these oils are highly unstable at high temperatures and the worst health choice for deep-fat frying was a message lost in translation. We were even encouraged to reuse previously heated oils (still a daily occurrence in most commercial kitchens and fast-food outlets), with each boiling of the oil creating ever more toxic compounds that cling tight to foods.

By the nineties, a scattering of studies started appearing in the academic journals revealing the startling level of damage these altered oils were doing, with the discovery that hydrogenation produces 'trans fats'. These man-made chemicals were being shown to be deadly for human health – dramatically increasing the risk for CHD, stroke and type 2 diabetes. At first, the food industry was largely in denial with a few notable exceptions – health campaigners such as myself and companies including Whole Earth, that launched Superspread in 1993. This prompted a complaint by the makers of Flora to the Advertising Standards Authority because Whole Earth said hydrogenated fat was bad for us. Interestingly, while they argued and appealed, Flora reduced their hydrogenated fat content from 21 per cent to less than 1 per cent.

However, the overwhelming strength of data was such that, by 2002, the US government had acknowledged that there is 'no safe limit' for trans fats – and that we should all therefore eat as little of it as possible (and in my view, none at all). Despite the health warnings on trans fats, in the form of partially hydrogenated vegetable oils, they still proliferate processed foods and are a big red flag for me on any food label. And although most processed seed oil spreads now proudly declare themselves to be trans-fat-free, I would still argue that eating butter is better, both for our health as well as for its taste (see page 116).

> **Make your own 'marg'**
> If you're wedded to the idea of using a soft-from-the-fridge spread, try making your own by whizzing together roughly equal quantities of olive oil with butter. Use basic olive oil, the less fancy (cheaper) version, as this has a blander taste more suitable to a spread than the more pungent extra-virgin olive oil. Simply blend the butter and oil together in a food processor and store in a tub in the fridge (it keeps for several weeks). This is a simple, healthier and more sustainable alternative to single-use plastic tubs of spreadable, butter-like gunk.

Spotlight on Fats and Oils

(*All fatty acid compositions are approximate and may vary according to their individual variety or origin, and butter depends on how cows have been fed.)

Animal fats

In days gone by, our grandmothers (or maybe great-grandmothers by now) would have cooked pretty much exclusively with lard, tallow or bacon drippings. These traditional fats are now coming back into vogue, as we start to realise their stability in cooking, great taste and many health benefits. But animal fat will only be as good as whatever the animal has eaten. Raised on grain or soya (which is most common), the fat will contain a significant amount of polyunsaturated fat. If an animal has been grazed on grass, these fats will contain more of the saturated and monounsaturated fats. So, if you're buying for health reasons, it makes sense to look for words such as 'grass-fed' or 'pasture-raised'.

You can also save your own drippings from meats. If you trim your meat before cooking, keep the fat for frying and save bacon drippings or any other kind of liquid fats for future use. I keep a small bowl in the fridge topped up with melted meat fats, ready to use for frying; cheaper than buying oil – it's also healthier and tastier too.

Butter
Saturated fat 68%, monounsaturated fat 28%, polyunsaturated fat 4%*

I use plenty of butter (both salted and unsalted, depending on what I fancy at the time) on a daily basis – and not only for its buttery, melt-in-the-mouth taste. Butter is nutritious as well as delicious. It's a naturally good source of fat-soluble nutrients such as vitamins A, E and K2, as well as selenium. It's also rich in the essential fatty acids conjugated linoleic acid (CLA) and butyrate, both real wellness warriors when it comes to nutrition. CLA is the form of fat that's been associated with brain health and shown to protect against weight gain, while butyrate is good for improving gut health and fighting inflammation in the body (butyrate supplements are popular for this reason). Butter also contains lecithin, a substance that assists with our cholesterol processing, among other fat-regulatory benefits.

The lowdown on ghee

Ghee (clarified butter) is also a good alternative for cooking as, when you clarify butter, you remove its lactose (milk sugars) and protein, leaving behind pure butterfat. It has a significantly higher smoke point than butter (250°C compared with 175°C for butter) making it a good option for frying.

Ghee is very easy to make:

- Pop some good-quality butter in a saucepan and simmer it over a low heat for 15–20 minutes without stirring until it has turned slightly brown (but not burnt) and the milk solids have risen to the top.
- Turn off the heat and leave to stand undisturbed as it cools.
- Line a sieve with a cloth or paper towel and carefully strain into a container, leaving the browned milk solids behind.

With milk solids and moisture removed, ghee will keep at room temperature for up to three months – and even longer if kept in the fridge.

Coconut oil

*Saturated fat 93%, monounsaturated fat 6%, polyunsaturated fat 1.6%**

If you don't mind the strong coconutty taste, coconut oil is a winner when it comes to cooking. It is highly saturated, so very stable when heated to high temperatures. It lasts for ages without refrigeration and also contains lauric acid, which has some interesting health benefits of its own, shown to improve cholesterol ratios (more on cholesterol in a moment) and can help kill bacteria and other bad bugs in the gut. The fats in coconut oil have also been shown to increase satiety (that nice feeling of fullness) and may even give the metabolism a bit of a boost.

Corn and other vegetable/seed oils
Saturated fat 14%, monounsaturated fat 42%, polyunsaturated fat 41%*

These are typically blended from several sources, such as sunflower, corn, rapeseed (canola), soya and safflower, so it's hard to be precise about its essential fatty acid profile as so much also depends on the refining process and which oils are blended together. But the bottom line is that all are high in the unstable, pro-inflammatory omega-6 fats (grapeseed is over 70 per cent polyunsaturates – possibly the most unstable of all). Corn oil is especially high in polyunsaturates and though its phytosterol and vitamin E contents may offer some health benefits, the view by some is that these are outweighted by the potential negative health effects. Interestingly, trans fats have also been detected in liquid vegetable/seed oils, as well as when they have been partially hydrogenated (see page 114).

Peanut oil has one of the highest smoke points (around 230°C) and is popular for frying as it has a neutral taste, but it is also high in polyunsaturates (around one third) making it prone to oxidative damage when heated. However, interestingly, peanut oil also contains resveratrol, a compound that helps fight heart disease and reduces cancer risk – I take a closer look at this longevity nutrient on page 289.

Macadamia nut oil
Saturated fat 5%, monounsaturated fat 87%, polyunsaturated fat 3%*

Mostly monounsaturated, similar to olive oil, this is a lovely light oil with a deliciously delicate flavour. However, it is very expensive so save it for high days and holidays if you fancy using it in the kitchen.

Olive oil

Saturated fat 14%, monounsaturated fat 75%, polyunsaturated fat 11%*

Olive oil is the king in the kitchen, being a versatile oil for frying, baking, salad dressings and just about everything else you can think of. Extra-virgin olive oil (often referred to as EVOO) is the first pressing of the olives and has the highest polyphenol content. It's also an excellent source of vitamins E and K2. It tends to be darker green in colour and has a much stronger, more pungent taste than 'pure' olive oil. The lighter and blander the olive oil, the more it will have been 'purified' to remove the active compounds. This happens as the olive mulch gets pressed and repressed to squeeze out every last drop of oil. Once the extra-virgin olive oil has been siphoned off, the remaining olive mixture is whizzed in a centrifuge to mechanically extract a bit more of the oil. After this, the traces of oil that still remain in the olive pulp are then extracted using chemical solvents. The more refined the oil, the paler and blander (and cheaper) it becomes.

I use pure or virgin olive oil for much of my cooking as it's less expensive and less flavourful, which is often what's needed in a recipe, but I always check the label to make sure it's not blended with a seed or vegetable oil. I mostly save my extra-virgin olive oil for drizzling onto veggies or for making salad dressings.

A 2018 study of 180 elderly people found that swapping out vegetable oil for a daily dose of extra-virgin olive oil improved brain function and memory recall after one year – perhaps one reason why those living in Mediterranean countries seem to have lower levels of dementia and Alzheimer's disease. In one 2007 study, extra-virgin olive oil was heated to 180°C for 36 hours and found to be highly resistant to damage, with a further 2017 review confirming that olive oil is comparable or better than other vegetable oils for frying at even higher temperatures (up to 190°C). It also has a similar smoke point to vegetable oils – around 200°C for olive oil compared to 205°C for blended vegetable oil. That said, I would still only ever heat any kind of oil once, which makes deep-fried foods an expensive rarity. Olive oil also has a high level of polyphenols, such as vitamin E and other phenolic compounds, that help prevent rancidity. Be aware that olive oil is subject to adulteration and false labelling. True extra-virgin olive oil turns slightly solid when placed in the fridge overnight – a simple and effective test for authenticity.

Palm oil

Saturated fat 50%, monounsaturated fat 40%, polyunsaturated fat 10%*

Obtained from the fruit of the oil palm, much has been said about the destructive nature of palm oil harvesting, as it has caused much deforestation and the removal of natural habitats for endangered creatures such as the orangutan. Sustainably sourced brands (from health food shops) are a good choice for cooking as palm oil is relatively stable at high temperatures. Red palm oil (which is unrefined) is also a useful source of vitamins E, co-enzyme Q10 and other fat-soluble nutrients.

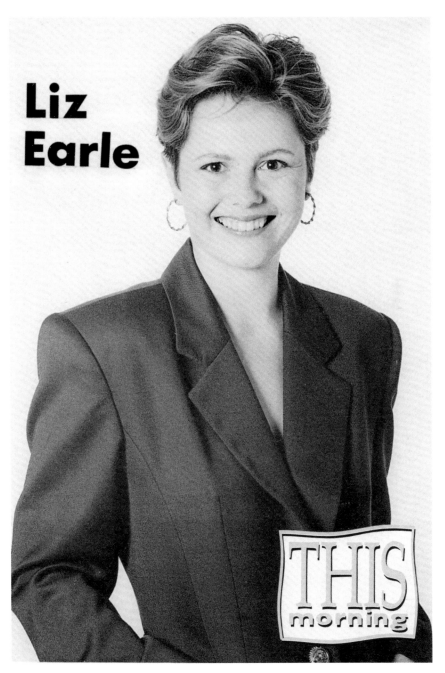

Liz Earle

My first TV job was on the launch of ITV's *This Morning* in 1988, ITV's flagship daytime show, where I was a contributor off and on for over thirty years.

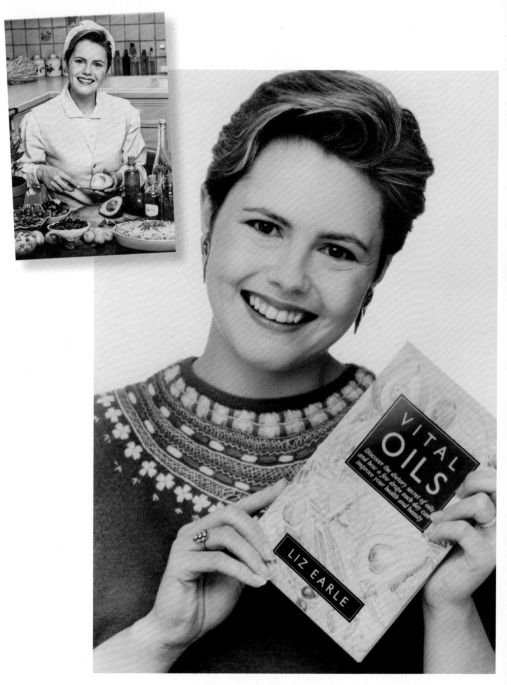

My first book, *Vital Oils*, was considered counter-cultural back in 1991 as it highlighted the importance of fats and oils at a time when low-fat was the general narrative.

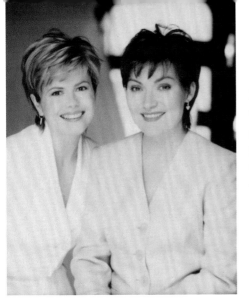

I've always loved working with Lorraine Kelly and sat to chat wellness and more on her studio sofa for many years during my time at GMTV.

This book accompanied my 1993 BBC TV series of the same name, Eat Yourself Beautiful, showing how what we eat can change how we look and feel.

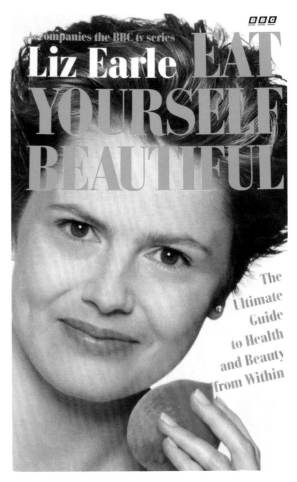

accompanies the BBC tv series

Liz Earle EAT YOURSELF BEAUTIFUL

The Ultimate Guide to Health and Beauty from Within

BBC

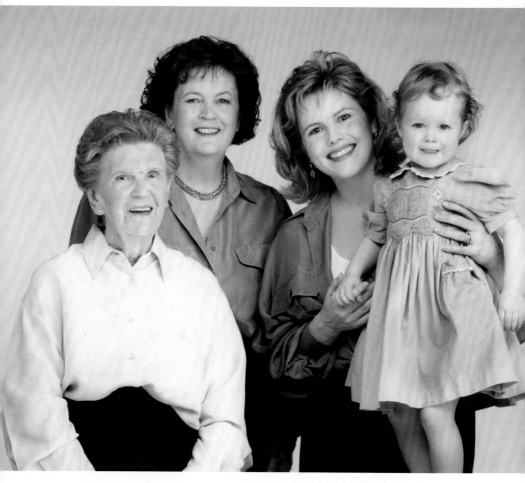

Four generations of the fabulous females in my family; my late Grandma Renee, my mother Ann, and my eldest child Amaryllis, better known as Lily, who was about two when this photo was taken for the *News of the World* magazine.

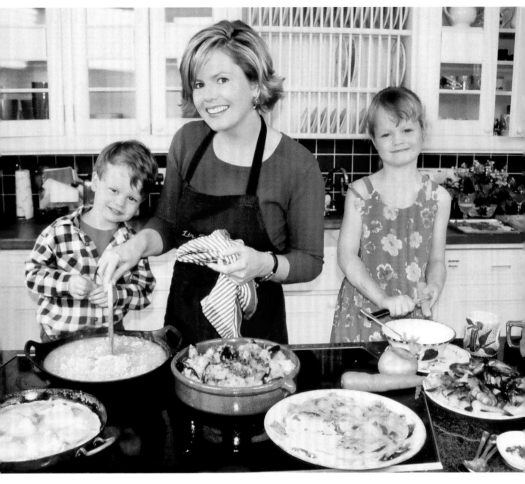

My two eldest children, Guy and Lily, would often appear on my afternoon TV show, *Liz Earle's Lifestyle,* which we filmed for three years in the 1990s at my London home in Putney.

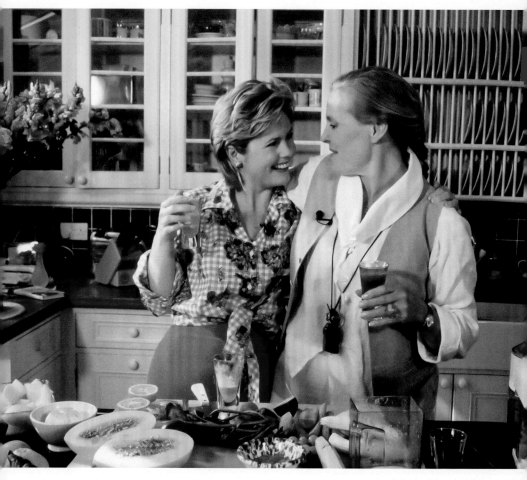

A highlight for me was when I interviewed the late Leslie Kenton on my TV show as she'd been such a strong influence for me in my early journalism career path.

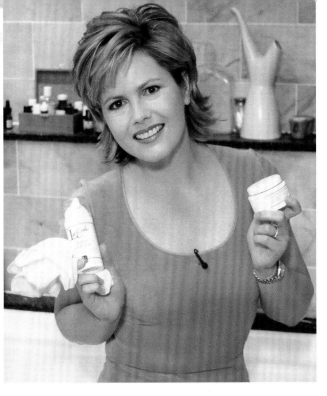

One of the first photos of me with my skincare line (note the original pink packaging!). We launched in 1995 and by the time my co-founder Kim and I sold in 2010, it had become one of the UK's biggest independent beauty brands.

I've always been a fan of eating eggs and this photo is from 1996 where I'm extolling their nutritional virtues for a TV segment on animal welfare and complete-protein foods.

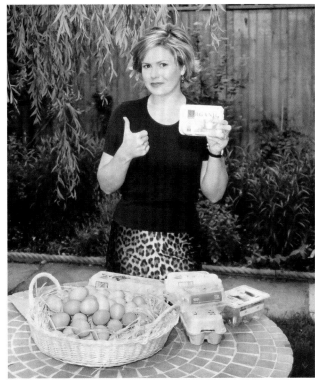

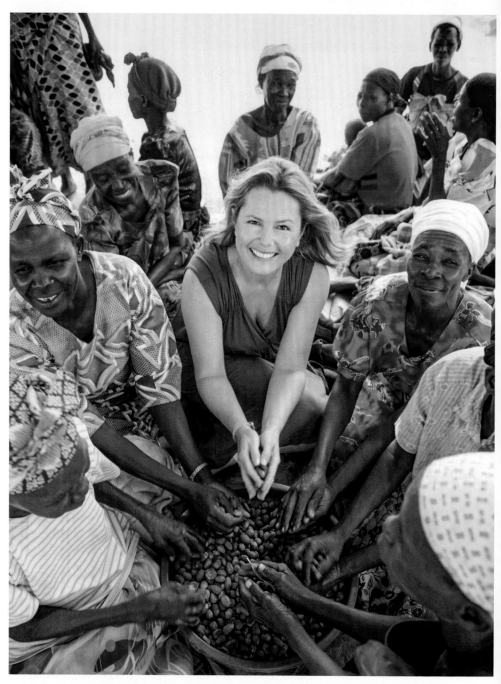

I travelled extensively during my time with Liz Earle Beauty Co., visiting many developing countries to find the best producers of botanical ingredients we could work with directly, such as this women's group in Southern Sudan producing shea nut oil.

Rapeseed oil

Saturated fat 7%, monounsaturated fat 52%, polyunsaturated fat 25%*

Also known as canola oil, especially in the US where the word 'rape' was rightly considered too off-putting for consumers when first introduced to the market. American rapeseed oil is solvent-extracted, highly processed using heat to maximise oil yield, contains trans fats and most likely to be GM-grown (genetically modified). All this has given canola/rapeseed a pretty bad name. Canola was also cross-bred to reduce the amount of erucic acid that gave original rapeseed oil a bitter taste. So, canola oil is essentially the highly processed, GM-version of rapeseed oil and, confusingly, here in the UK, the term canola or rapeseed can be interchanged.

There's been a surge in the number of British farmers who now grow rapeseed for oil, with many smaller, niche brands proudly declaring themselves to be 'cold-pressed', locally and sustainably grown. So, is it a good alternative to olive oil? Well, it's certainly cheaper, and cold-pressed avoids traces of chemical solvent and trans fats in the oil (although cold-pressing is a bit of a misnomer, as heat is generated in the process so it's not entirely cold). Rapeseed does have a very strong flavour though, which is why the processed form of rapeseed oil is more popular with both consumers and the food industry. Rapeseed oil has a high smoke point of around 450°C and, thanks to those double bonds (see page 123), it can be considered a good alternative to olive oil for frying. However, intensive rapeseed mono-cropping needs high inputs of pesticides and fertilisers, and is usually highly processed, so unless a rapeseed oil is organically grown (at the time of writing there is just one Yorkshire grower), I would have to say that, overall, it possibly carries more harms than benefits when compared to olive oil.

In order of preference in my kitchen, I use olive oil, lard, ghee/butter, coconut oil and organic rapeseed oil, sometimes with a splash of macadamia or avocado oil too. I use lard for frying, beef dripping or poultry fat for roasting potatoes and occasionally coconut oil, for recipes that can carry its distinctive flavour (such as Thai or Chinese dishes).

When it comes to cooking, switching out vegetable/seed oils for traditional, healthy mono- and/or saturated fats is probably one of the simplest, healthiest food swaps we can make.

Whichever oil you end up using, it's important to protect it from the factors that cause oxidation: heat, air and light. Always store in a cool, dark place and put the lid back on as soon as you've used it. Buying smaller amounts that get used up more quickly is more expensive but better than a bulk buy.

The Different Types of Fats and Oils

It's easy to feel flummoxed by the many different types of fats and oils and their various health harms or benefits, but in chemical terms, it all boils down to their double bonds. Fats and oils fall into different categories depending on how many double bonds their chemical structure contains. Saturated fats don't have any (they are 'full', i.e. saturated); monounsaturated have one double bond (hence 'mono' meaning single); and polyunsaturated fats have two or more double bonds. The more double bonds a fat or oil has, the less stable it is and the more prone it is to oxidation (going rancid). This process of oxidation happens both on the supermarket shelf and, more worryingly, inside our bodies. If we have a lot of unstable fats in our diets (such as polyunsaturates), there's a strong chance our cell membranes are going to be more sensitive to oxidation and inflammation. This is why we're hearing increasing talk about vegetable/seed oils being pro-inflammatory and something to be avoided in foods.

Saturated (mostly solid at room temperature)
- Coconut oil
- Dairy (cheese, cream)
- Egg yolks
- Palm oil
- Meats

Monounsaturated (omega-9s)
- Chicken, goose and duck fat
- Lard
- Olive oil
- Rapeseed (canola) oil

Polyunsaturated (omega-6s)
- Corn oil
- Cottonseed oil
- Peanut oil
- Safflower oil
- Soya bean oil
- Sunflower oil

Polyunsaturated (omega-3s)
Also polyunsaturated, these oils have their last double bond in a different place on the carbon atom chain, making them act differently (and more healthily) in the body.
- Evening primrose and starflower/borage oil
- Fish oils (for example, cod liver oil, fish oil and krill supplements)
- Flax seed

Partially hydrogenated vegetable oils
These oils have been hardened and contain damaging trans fats.
- Many baked goods
- Most biscuits
- Crisps
- Margarine

The '3-6-9 ratio'

When turning the spotlight on the health properties of oils, many nutritionists will refer to the '3-6-9 ratio'. This refers to the amount and type of omega fatty acids an oil contains – and is an important reference.

Omega-3

Omega-3s have become well known as being the healthier fats, found in fish oils, and include EPA and DHA (see page 105), as well as alpha-linolenic acid (ALA). They are especially important in midlife and beyond, and play a critical role in our brain chemistry, as well as helping with weight management, reducing liver fats and fighting general cell inflammation. I'll be taking a closer look at these on page 227 in relation to fish oil supplements and brain health.

Omega-6

Omega-6s are found in vegetable and seed oils. A small amount of omega-6 is essential, but too much tips the balance towards ill health. Too high a level in our daily diets increases our risk of inflammation and inflammatory disease. Despite their commercial monopoly, more studies are seeping into the mainstream around the safety of omega-6 seed oils, with concern about their pro-inflammatory effects, especially when it comes to brain health and ageing. Omega-6 polyunsaturates have also shown a strong link with promoting tumours, notably breast cancer (by contrast, omega-3 fats from fish oils have been shown to be cancer-protective, especially for colon and breast cancers). There are a couple of exceptions here worth a mention:

evening primrose oil and borage (starflower seed) oil, both rich in GLA, which although not readily eaten in foods, can be a very helpful oil supplement to take for certain inflammatory conditions, including eczema. CLA is another omega-6 fatty acid linked to several health benefits, including fat loss.

Omega-9

The last remaining category is the omega-9s, or monounsaturated oils such as olive oil and, to a lesser extent, rapeseed oil. Studies consistently show health benefits from these, including reduced cell inflammation and better insulin sensitivity.

The key is eating the right ratio of omega-3, -6 and -9 essential fatty acids, which nutritionists advise as 2:1:1. Unfortunately, most modern Western diets rely very heavily on omega-6 from refined vegetable and seed oils, which tips the balance away from health benefits into health damage, and moves the ratio closer to 1:6:1. In order to live long and age well, we should be focusing far more on the omega-3s and -9s.

Cholesterol Concerns

If saturated fats are not the dietary baddie we've been led to believe, where does that leave cholesterol? Surely that must play a supporting role somewhere here when it comes to raising risk factors for CHD and stroke? Well, again, the short answer is no. The longer answer is, of course, more nuanced. Cholesterol *does* play a role, but perhaps not the one we might think. Cholesterol is a natural substance, made in the body by the liver. It's fundamentally important for good health. Without cholesterol we would die. We couldn't be cholesterol-free even if we wanted to be, as our bodies simply manufacture their own when supplies from our diets get low. In fact, only about 20 per cent of our total cholesterol levels come from food (one reason why restricting cholesterol-rich foods, such as eggs, is such nonsense). Cholesterol is the starting point for many key hormones, including oestrogen, progesterone and testosterone (our HRT holy trinity), so I especially advocate *against* a low-fat diet in our middle years and beyond. In addition, cholesterol helps with the production of bile acids (which aid digestion) and the absorption of fat-soluble vitamins such as vitamin D, essential for strong bones and a healthy immune function.

In order to get to where it's needed in the body, cholesterol needs a form of transport, and this is where the lipoproteins come in. Operating a bit like a taxi service, low-density lipoproteins (LDLs – the so-called 'bad' cholesterol) carry cholesterol around the body, whereas high-density lipoproteins (HDLs – the 'good' cholesterol) absorb the remainder and return back to the liver for processing. Controlling our cholesterol levels, specifically the ratio between our HDL and LDL, has been a major public health message for the prevention of heart disease. GPs carry out finger-prick blood tests to assess our levels of 'good' and 'bad' blood fats, and often go on to prescribe statins to anyone over the age of 60 (or even younger). The most lucrative drug in medical history, statins are now prescribed to well over a billion people around the globe. The vested interest in sustaining the statin narrative for wellbeing is vast (and vocal). Unfortunately, there is little evidence that statins have resulted in a big reduction of death rates from heart disease – and many report unwelcome side effects including muscle aches and extreme fatigue (most likely linked to the depletion of co-enzyme Q 10, as discussed on page 65). Another component of cholesterol that routinely gets measured is triglyceride levels. These are the main constituents of body fat and are fundamental in converting glucose into energy.

To assess the impact of all this, in 1948 a major US health study was launched called the Framingham Heart Study (FHS). It is used the world over as the basis for all medical-school training when teaching doctors how to assess a patient's risk of developing heart disease. The FHS looked at various factors, including smoking, high blood pressure, high cholesterol and type 2 diabetes. These top four factors still drive medical doctrine today. However, while very high levels of cholesterol (affecting less than 10 per cent of the overall population) may well be a serious risk factor, for the vast majority of us (over 90 per cent, in fact), cholesterol was not even slightly significant. Even the American Heart Association says that cholesterol in food is a 'nutrient of non-concern'. This is a pretty astonishing finding, when you consider how much dietary and prescription advice is based on this one, potentially flawed, premise.

One of the lead authors involved with the FHS study, Dr William Castelli, published a review of its findings in 1996. He noted that unless LDL levels were very high (above 7.8mmol/L or >3,000mg/dL) they were of no value in isolation in predicting the risk of heart disease. It is the total cholesterol to HDL ratio that is the most predictive of heart disease, not total cholesterol levels. Interestingly, for every 1mg/dl drop in cholesterol per year, there was a 14 per cent *increase* in cardiovascular death and an 11 per cent increase in the following 18 years for those aged 50 and over. Subsequent studies show that, for older people, higher LDL cholesterol levels may actually be heart-protective. Further analysis by public health researcher

Dr Zoe Harcombe PhD, a favourite guest of mine on my podcast, has also shown that higher total cholesterol levels are actually associated with a lower risk of death. Writing in the *New England Journal of Medicine* as long ago as 1977, the medical research professor George Mann wrote an excoriating review contending that evidence of diet-heart connection was inconclusive at best and wholly incorrect at worst. After he retired from medicine, Mann proclaimed that the demonising of saturated fat was 'the greatest scam in the history of medicine'. So where does this leave us now, other than confused?

A discussion with your GP may well result in further confusion, as despite this analysis of World Health Organization (WHO) published data, the cut-off for a 'healthy' cholesterol score on the charts supplied to GPs has actually been lowering over the years. Of course, as the official threshold is lowered, so the prescribing of lucrative anti-cholesterol medications increases and the narrative intensifies. There is no doubt that the build-up of fatty deposits inside our arteries form plaques that can become larger, may block arteries and lead to heart attacks. The question, though, is whether LDL is the cholesterol-carrying culprit – or if there is some other, more suspicious suspect.

A major review published in the *Journal of Food and Nutrition Research* called 'Food consumption and the actual statistics of cardiovascular diseases: an epidemiological comparison of 42 European countries' found 'Our results do not support the association between CVDs [cardiovascular diseases] and saturated fat, which is still contained in dietary guidelines. Instead, they agree with data accumulated from studies that link CVD risk with the high glycaemic index/load of carbohydrate-based diets'. So if eating high-fat foods doesn't actually lead to fatty deposits building up in our arteries, as would seem logical, then what does?

Inflammation and blood clotting

Arterial plaque is made up of deposits of oxidised LDL cholesterol, inflammatory or immune system cells and calcium. The latest thinking is that a build-up of plaque is triggered by chronic inflammation, caused by a number of varying factors. However, it is not the furring up of our arteries itself that is the killer, but the formation of a blood clot within a narrowed artery. Perhaps it would be more helpful to look at heart disease as a problem more to do with inflammation and blood clotting. Smoking (and passive smoking) is a significant factor, along with environmental pollution, as both increase platelet activity, making blood thicker, stickier and more likely to clot. High blood pressure is also a significant factor, likely caused by insulin resistance (when our bodies don't respond properly to the insulin the body makes). And type 2 diabetes, where the body is unable to keep blood-glucose levels stable, also makes the blood more likely to clot. Better control of our blood glucose spikes is a key part of better metabolic health and more likely to be the best way to reduce overall heart disease, which leads me neatly on to the question of carbs.

The Case Against Carbs

Most of us tend to think of carbohydrates as coming from bread, rice, pasta, sugary buns and the like, but in fact, carbohydrate is present in almost all foods, including fruit and veg. *Any* form of carbohydrate that we eat ends up as glucose in the bloodstream. Some forms get in there more quickly than others and cause a rapid destabilising spike in blood sugar (such as potatoes, white rice, any kind of corn and refined flours), followed by the energy crash as levels swiftly slump. Others are what are known as 'slow-release'

Five ways to lower your blood pressure

Healthy blood pressure is below 120 over 80 mm Hg. Above 140/80 is considered to be high. Home blood pressure monitors are a cheap and simple way to check.

1. Aerobic and resistance exercise both lower blood pressure as they strengthen the heart muscle so it needs less effort to pump blood around, reducing stress on arteries and lowering blood pressure.
2. Maintaining a healthy weight and shifting excess body fat reduces blood pressure. Cutting back on sugar and carbs helps here.
3. Getting plenty of potassium in the diet helps reduce inflammation in the blood vessels. Good foods for this include milk and yoghurt, veggies, bananas, lentils and beans. Upping protein levels can also help lower blood pressure.
4. Don't smoke! The chemicals in tobacco narrow the arteries and cause inflammation, increasing blood pressure.
5. Manage stress levels with deep breathing, listening to soothing music, taking a walk in nature and meditation.

carbs, as they convert into glucose more slowly, for example, brown rice, which is slowed by its additional fibre content.

Carbs are always made up of sugars, and there are many kinds. Technically, there are three main groups: single, double and multi, similar to the many different types of fats and oils (see pages 123–6). Single sugars are monosaccharides and these include glucose, fructose and galactose. The double-sugars are sucrose, lactose and maltose. The polysaccharides or many-sugars split into two types: soluble and insoluble/indigestible, which include highly fibrous foods (such as bran).

According to the Institute of Medicine (US) Panel on Macronutrients 2005, 'the lower limit of dietary carbohydrate compatible with life apparently is zero'. In other words, the human body does not actually need *any* carbohydrate and we can survive without it.

The question of fibre

Fibrous foods such as oats, brown rice, wholewheat flour and the like are very low in important nutrients, such as vitamins A, C, D, E and K as well as the B-complex vitamins. Technically, we have no nutritional requirement for highly fibrous foods such as grains and bran. However, we do know that our good gut bugs thrive on insoluble fibre such as inulin and GOS/FOS, found in pre and probiotics (more on page 214), and I am a fan of these. Some of the more extreme proponents of the zero-sugar brigade don't actually eat any fibre at all, such as those following the 'carnivore diet'. This involves living on meat, fish and eggs. As I say, this is at the extreme end, but advocates cite a carnivore diet as being helpful for some debilitating health conditions, such as chronic autoimmune issues, fibromyalgia, migraine, epilepsy, rheuma-toid arthritis, ankylosing spondylitis and the like. This kind of no-sugar eating puts the body into a state of ketosis, where it burns ketones instead of glucose for energy. It's at the hardcore end of high-fat, low-carb eating and is sometimes used by func-tional medicine practitioners to help hard-to-treat illness when other strategies have failed. I know of several people who have been helped by this way of eating, even as a temporary fix to 'reset' the system. It's worth investigating if you think this might be something you could benefit from and I have included some useful links and contacts on page 307 for further guidance.

Anti-nutrients

Vegans, vegetarians and non-meat-eaters tend to eat a much more carbohydrate-dense diet, getting much of their protein and daily nutrition from pulses, nuts, seeds and beans. However, when it comes to grains, pulses and legumes (such as beans, split peas and lentils), there's been more recent talk about the negative effects of their phytate content on the body. Phytates or phytic acid in whole grains, seeds, legumes and some nuts can leach important minerals such as zinc, iron, magnesium and calcium from our systems. Legumes and whole grains also contain saponins, which decrease the absorption of important nutrients. Saponins are triterpene glycosides, most commonly found in soya beans, chickpeas, quinoa, peanuts and spinach. They are the plants' natural defence mechanism to ward off bacterial disease and stop them being devoured by pests. Naturally slightly toxic to protect against predators, the word comes from the Latin 'sapo' meaning soap, as they have a slightly foamy characteristic (you may have noticed this when opening a can of chickpeas – the bubbly 'aquafaba' is filled with saponins). Although poisonous to insects, snails, fish and the like, that toxicity is not thought to carry over to human health as saponins are broken down by our digestive enzymes. As with anything though, we are all individual, and some may react differently to these phytochemicals than others, so it's good to be aware of what *might* be causing any digestive issues.

Phytates, saponins and lectins have all been described as 'anti-nutrients' as they reduce nutrient availability, and high levels are linked to intestinal damage and inflammation. However, the jury is out on whether there is enough hard evidence to cut them out of our diets altogether. If you are clinically anaemic (low in iron) or at risk of osteoporosis (requiring plenty of calcium), it is worth being aware of these minerals being depleted, especially if you are a plant-based eater. To reduce the phytate, saponin and lectin content of plant foods, simply soak them overnight before eating. This is one reason why 'overnight oats' are more easily digested than muesli. Adding a splash of cider vinegar for extra glucose-reducing properties is also helpful in breaking down unwanted compounds, and cooking also reduces the anti-nutrient load (cooked porridge is likely to be better for us than raw wheatgerm or oatmeal, for example). Sourdoughing of breads also helps reduce the phytate content. In fact, soaking, cooking or fermenting makes all kinds of carbohydrates more digestible and user-friendly. I definitely include some of these in my daily diet, as I personally find the compelling evidence for fibre involves its role in feeding our beneficial gut bugs with something called resistant starch. This is the form of insoluble fibre that we don't digest but which is good for our good gut bacteria to graze on, enabling them to multiply. However, as I've gotten older, I tend to follow the 80:20 rule when it comes to carbs (20 per cent being my rough daily guide) and generally stick to a low-carb, high-fat and protein diet. Of course, I'll have that slice of birthday cake or square of chocolate (more of which later), but I've found the fewer carbs I eat, the less I crave them. And that's no bad thing.

Protein Power

Alongside healthy fats and fewer carbs, I'm also a big believer in eating more protein, a fundamental building block for better physical and mental health. Replacing at least some of the carbs in our daily diets with good sources of protein increases fat loss, especially

Timing matters

Some of the most interesting dietary research is now looking at not only what foods we eat, but the order in which we eat them. Eating vegetables, fats and protein before eating carbohydrates has been shown to lower glucose levels, reduce insulin spikes and decrease insulin sensitivity. For me, this means a boiled egg for breakfast before any toast or cereal, and I eat some green veggies and protein before any rice or potatoes in meals. A simple switch around of the foods we eat can make a big difference when it comes to weight loss too. This is because keeping our blood-sugar levels stable is so helpful, warding off hunger pangs, controlling sugar-fix food cravings and preventing the onset of type 2 diabetes (an ever-growing and very serious health concern). So instead of dieticians telling us 'don't eat that' the advice should be more along the lines of 'eat this, then eat that . . .', says Dr Louis Aronne, professor of metabolic research and clinical medicine at Weill Cornell medical college in the United States.

around the tummy (great for combatting 'middle-age spread'). It also eliminates food cravings, gives our metabolism a helpful boost and helps us recover lean tissue and build stronger muscles. I've become even more aware of its importance as we age and now make some kind of protein source the mainstay of every meal, and then build around this. For example, I'll have a couple of boiled eggs for breakfast with a few chopped-up carrot sticks on the side – and then a slice of sourdough toast spread with butter, avocado, Marmite or almond butter (but rarely marmalade or jam). I love a nice slice of white bread, thickly spread with homemade strawberry jam, but this is an occasional treat, not an everyday go-to. If I do eat toast and jam, I'll make sure I've first fuelled up with a few healthy fats and protein (such as eggs or a nice thick, plain yoghurt) so as not to spike my insulin levels by eating a load of sugary foods on an otherwise empty stomach. Those with high blood pressure or type 2 diabetes have also been shown to have improved blood-sugar control when eating more protein in their diets.

So how much protein is the right amount for us to age well? Many sports medics and nutritionists advocate three to four 30–50g protein servings a day if you are looking to change your body composition and shape i.e. lose wobbly fat and build stronger muscle tone. This is a higher level of protein than most of us would eat on a regular basis, but can help shift us towards a leaner, more toned shape and is the kind of level needed if we're spending more time working out (especially resistance training or high-intensity, which I'll cover in Chapter 9). More doesn't always mean better. Current data suggests that 40–60g is the maximum amount of protein that can be used by the body for muscle synthesis in any one sitting. As a general rule, aim for a palm-sized amount of protein on your plate (so, the bigger you are, the more you need). Plant-based eaters can opt for protein-rich tofu, tempeh and other soya-derived foods. Soya beans (edamame) are a favourite of mine as they're not only rich in gut-bug-boosting dietary fibre, but are also an excellent source of plant protein. Frozen edamame are one of my basic freezer foods! Pulses such as dried peas and lentils, legumes and beans are also good sources of 'incomplete' protein (albeit with higher levels of anti-nutrients), meaning that they have some, but not all, of the nine essential amino acids we can only obtain from the food we eat, all found in animal proteins. For example, chickpeas contain most of the amino acids, but lack sulphur-containing methionine and cystine (depending on which data you go by). Note: all beans and pulses should be soaked and well cooked before eating to reduce their anti-nutrient content. Rice is also a useful protein source, but is missing lysine, which is why plant-based combinations are so important for those not eating animal protein. Good examples include rice and beans, chickpeas and wheat (such as hummus on sourdough), an almond butter sandwich or pasta and peas. I'm also a fan of a handful of almonds as a healthy high-protein snack. It's not as good as a slice of cheese and is lacking in the amino acid lysine, but a handful contains around 6g protein (as well as prebiotic 'insoluble' fibre, which keeps me feeling fuller for longer and less likely to reach for a Twix . . .).

A word about protein powders

One of the easiest ways to top up our protein supplies is with a scoop of protein powder added to a shake, smoothie or yoghurt – and even to home cooking such as porridge, scrambled eggs, pancakes and muffins. There are many different types on the market, from dairy to hemp and even insects, such as crickets. They all provide some form of protein, but all are slightly different. Two that have stood the test of time come from milk and they are whey and casein proteins. Both are high-quality 'complete' proteins, containing all nine of the essential amino acids we need for health.

Casein protein is considered superior to whey as it is absorbed more slowly by the body, providing protein at a slower, steadier rate so we feel fuller for longer, making it ideal for intermittent fasting (see page 174) or for having in the evening before bed. Whey protein is absorbed and used by the body much more quickly, which is why it's good to take before and after an intense workout.

Some sources of protein

Food	Protein per 100g
Chicken breast	32.0g
Beef steak	31.0g
Lamb chop	29.2g
Tuna and salmon	24.9g
Cheddar cheese	25.4g
Almonds*	21.1g
Mackerel	20.3g
Crab (tinned)	18.1g
Oysters	18.0g
Prawns	15.4g
Eggs	14.7g
Walnuts*	14.7g
Wholewheat such as bread*	12.2g
White rice*	10.9g
Cottage cheese	9.4g
Tofu*	8.1g
Bread*	7.9g
Red lentils*	7.6g
Chickpeas*	7.2g
Greek-style yoghurt	5.7g
Baked beans*	5.0g
Skimmed milk	3.5g
Whole milk	3.4g
Soya milk (plain)*	2.4g
Oat milk*	1.0g
Almond milk*	0.4g

Source: McCance and Widdowson's *The Composition of Foods* (Royal Society of Chemistry, 2015)

* Plant-based sources are all incomplete protein i.e. lacking one or more essential amino acid – see above.

Whey protein contains more of the branched-chain amino acids (BCAAs) leucine, isoleucine and valine, while casein contains a higher proportion of the amino acids histadine, methionine and phenylananine. Casein also contains helpful peptides needed for a healthy immune system and digestive system. These peptides are also heart-healthy as they help lower blood pressure and reduce the formation of blood clots, as well as improving the absorption of calcium and phosphorus. By contrast, whey protein includes immunoglobulins that support our immune systems and can help kill off harmful viruses and bacteria. They also improve our absorption of vitamin A and iron.

There are also plant-based sources of protein powder, such as pea protein, also known as pea protein isolate as it's made by isolating the protein part of yellow peas to make a beige-coloured powder. Pea protein is unusual for a plant food as it contains all nine of the essential amino acids, although it's relatively low in methionine. Like whey, it's a good source of the BCAAs, although milk-derived protein powders do tend to be more easily absorbed by the body. Pea protein has had a bit of a bad press in recent years with the discovery that some brands contain high levels of glyphosate (pesticide) residues. In 2022, the Clean Label Project, a non-profit group in America, also reported finding traces of heavy metals (lead, arsenic, cadmium and mercury) in some vegan brands, additionally discovered by the supplement testing website Consumerlab.com. Out of 134 top-selling protein powder brands tested by the Clean Label Project, those sourced from eggs came out 'cleanest' with plant-based protein sources revealed as being the worst (with 75 per cent of plant-based samples testing positive for lead). Another plant-based protein is hemp, rich in omega-3 essential fatty acids (although their conversion to beneficial EPA/

DHA brain fats is limited). It is also not considered a 'complete' protein as it has very low levels of lysine and leucine, so is not an ideal source.

In terms of which one to use as a protein supplement, I would consider casein first for weight loss, with additional whey protein for those stepping up their exercise regime or wanting to put on muscle tone more quickly. Pea protein isolate is a reasonable alternative for those who prefer to be dairy-free. One scoop of casein or whey protein powder yields around 24–28g pure protein. Pea protein isolate contains around 15–20g pure protein per scoop. As a precaution, always buy plant-based protein powders from a well-established, reputable brand and check out their safety data and toxicity testing credentials online before purchasing. I also like unflavoured bone broth powder as a source of high quality protein (around 90g per 100g, or 18g per average scoop).

Why I Changed My Mind About Meat

As a wellness writer, I'm sometimes asked why I'm not a vegan, or even a vegetarian. Once upon a time, I was a macrobiotic vegan, balancing my 'yin and yang' on a plate, living on miso soup, brown rice and seaweed. I gave it up after a year or so as I started to feel unwell and found it to be highly antisocial. We're talking about 30 years ago, when there were few places to eat outside the home and I was viewed with extreme suspicion at eighties' dinner parties, where I'd bring my own food box. Fast forward several decades and what I eat now could not be more different.

A few years ago, my then-husband and I ran one of the UK's first grass-fed regenerative pasture farms. We were a founding farm for

Pasture for Life, an organisation that supports grazed animals on the land as a way of rearing healthier meat and dairy, as well as regenerating the soil's all-important microbiome and capturing carbon. Cows are often demonised in the media as being a significant contributor to climate change. This may be true of the vast feed lots across middle America, where millions of animals are kept on arid soil, exclusively fed on GM soya and grains (although their contribution to 'global warming', such as it might be, is extraordinarily small compared to intensive crop agriculture and factory food production, especially ultra-processed foods like fake meat). This is a very different picture to the way the majority of animals live here in the UK, a landscape historically dominated for thousands of years by pastoral grazing. The methane cycle of cows kept on grasslands actually sequesters or traps carbon, locking it into the soil. Naturally grazing animals are a vital part of a healthy ecosystem and are beneficial for the planet – a seemingly inconvenient fact too often overlooked by statisticians, who for some unknown reason seem to base their findings only on intensively reared, US feed-lot animals.

Grazing animals, such as those in the UK and much of Europe, are fundamental for a sustainable, more natural, form of food production.

Grazing animals are essential for maintaining top soil, preventing soil erosion and building soil fertility; a farming system that is not only healthier for us, but also significantly better for our planet.

I'm going to leave the ethical debate of meat-eating to one side, as this is a book about healthspan and longevity and not moral philosophy. When studying the data, remember there are 'lies, damned lies and statistics', to quote Mark Twain (and the cultivation of plant foods kills millions of pollinators and smaller mammals in the process).

It's important to remember that not all foods classed as 'meat' are equal. You don't need me to tell you that there's a world of difference between an industrially processed meat pie and a simple piece of grilled steak, especially if that steak comes from a grass-fed or 'pastured' cow, raised on grass and not grain or soya. Yet the statisticians and researchers in this area, sometimes funded by vested interests, seem to base the majority of their studies on all 'meat' products, putting the health risks or benefits of, say, a Spam sandwich in the same category as a piece of sirloin. Even the NHS website lumps the two together, giving its guidelines on eating 'red and processed meats', as if the two were the same. To me, that is about as sensible as advising how much 'broccoli and buns' we should be eating. This is how anti-meat headlines are created, why meat so often falls to the bottom of any 'health-food' list and even gets banned from some school and university cafeterias, out of the reach of developing brains that truly need high-quality animal produce the most.

The difference between the types of meat you may (or may not) choose to eat is important. Pastured meat has a lower saturated fat content, higher levels of important omega-3 fatty acids and a lower, more balanced (healthier) ratio of omega-6 to omega-3 fatty acids (see page 125). Remember this: it's not what *we* eat that matters so much as what what we eat has eaten. An animal grazed on grass will produce food (meat or dairy) that has a different nutritional profile from one raised on GM soya and grain, so grass-fed beef or lamb is preferable to grain-fed chicken or pork. In particular, pastured meat (and dairy products such as milk and cheese) contains higher levels of CLA (see page 116). Meat and dairy from animals raised on pasture also have higher vitamin and mineral levels than those foods from grain-fed animals, notably the fat-soluble vitamins A and E, and minerals such as calcium, magnesium and potassium. Meat even contains antioxidants too, which is interesting as we tend to think we only get these nutrients from plants.

Animal welfare is obviously a very important concern and pasture-fed livestock live their natural lives outdoors, feeding on pasture and forage, such as hay (dried grass called haylage) during the winter. Studies show they're less likely to suffer from disease and require little veterinary attention or antibiotics when compared to intensively reared livestock, especially where animals are cooped up indoors. I remember having a financial audit many years ago when I was involved with organic farming and the accountant asking where all our missing vet bills were. 'We don't have any,' I replied. So, pasture-based is better for us and better for the animals, but also significantly better for the environment too. The carbon footprint of grass farms is significantly lower than that of farms where cereal crops are grown to feed animals (or humans). Visit any organic or regenerative grass-based farm and you'll also find a much richer biodiversity of wild flowers, pollinating insects and nesting habitats for birds and small mammals. For all these reasons, it's important to read food labels carefully (see page 159 for more tips on this) and buy less, better-quality meat and dairy (which works out to be the same cost in the long run).

In recent years, the commercial interests of the food industry have driven us into buying plant-based and ultra-processed foods (UPFs) and scared us away from traditional agriculture – good for business, where 'plant-based' could refer to the industrial plants that produce them, but not for our health.

**Food choices can be complicated and I
can't help but wonder if the food industry
sets out to cause deliberate confusion,
just so we give up and have a snack!**

The reality of junk food

What we choose to feed our bodies with on a daily basis is the biggest health intervention we can make. Simply making the decision to add in more of the good stuff will help crowd out the unhelpful diet destroyers. Recognise that fast food, UPFs and pretty much anything out of a packet is produced for profit, certainly not for your personal wellbeing. You are being sold to – manipulated by advertising and deliberately addicted to processed foods by the cunning use of very specific habit-forming ingredients including clever sugar-salt-fat combinations and synthetic flavouring agents, added to make food almost impossible to stop eating.

Researchers in Germany recently published a study showing that some flavourings added to foods (be they 'natural' or artificial flavours) promote over-eating by switching off the body's appetite control mechanism. These lab flavourings appear to bypass our natural feelings of fullness so gluttony takes over. Clever food engineering creates processed foods with 'hyperpalatability' in mind to also keep us eating it. Fat, sugar and salt mixtures activate our brain–reward neurocircuits in the same way as drugs like cocaine, which is why we love them so much. Recognise this and you'll realise that it's time to break the junk-food cycle, step off the hamster wheel and regain control of your mind, body – and budget.

Milk and Dairy Matters

The debate around milk – good or bad? – has become a bit of a hot potato, to mix food metaphors. Let's first explore the myth of milk as being inflammatory, one of the most common criticisms I hear when talking about cow's milk. Looking at the widest body of evidence, in the form of three systematic reviews (which pull together all the research studies for the overall big picture, to give the most accurate analysis), these show that dairy foods have either no effect on inflammation or a positive benefit. Are you surprised? These reviews do cover all kinds of dairy foods, including milk, cheese and fermented dairy such as yoghurt and kefir, so it's hard to drill down into the precise data on each, but it is pretty clear that there seems to be little general correlation between eating dairy produce and inflammation. However, I should point out that we're all different and our gut bacteria are likely to play an important role in how we react to dairy.

In terms of the role of our gut bacteria, some studies suggest that milk increases mucus levels, while others show that milk does not increase mucus, but that it may affect the texture of it in the body and how we sense it, so could make us more mucus-aware. This may be due to changes to our gut lining permeability, so it's likely our gut bacteria are at work here and not the actual foods that we're eating causing an individual reaction.

For any kind of food intolerance, it's important to look at the 'me-search' instead of the re-search. Our own bodies can reveal more personally useful information than any study. Some may be sensitive to the A1 gene in milk, a modern gene-type now common in dairy production. To test this, those who react to cow's milk can try A2 milk, as many of those who consider themselves to be lactose intolerant can actually handle A2 milk without any issues. Whether a cow produces A1 or A2 milk depends on genetics – some breeds have a higher proportion of A2 genes within their population, for example, Guernsey. It's worth looking for Guernsey milk, or milk specifically labelled as coming from A2 cows, if this might be helpful for you. Understanding and listening to our own bodies is vital – so much more so than dismissing an important and nutritious group of foods on the basis of a hand-picked study promoted to financially benefit others. If you can tolerate real milk, my personal view is that it is a healthy choice.

Lactose versus casein intolerance

A true food allergy affects the immune system and can trigger severe symptoms, including anaphylaxis and death. Allergies can be genetic and we still don't fully understand what causes them, although those with a history of allergic conditions such as hay fever, asthma and eczema are more vulnerable. By contrast, a food intolerance often affects only the digestive system and causes less serious symptoms. They are often caused by a faulty digestive system and may develop when our gut health is damaged.

A casein allergy is when the body mistakenly identifies casein as a dangerous threat and triggers an immune response to fight it off. Most common in young bottle-fed babies, most who have a casein allergy will have outgrown it by the time they reach five years of age. This is different from a lactose intolerance which happens when we don't produce enough of the enzyme lactase in order to digest lactose, the sugar found in milk, causing gas and digestive bloating. Lactose intolerance is often genetic and is most common in those of Asian, African and South American origin. It can be overcome by taking enzyme supplements before eating any foods or drinks containing lactose (most lactose-free brands don't actually remove the lactose, they simply add the lactose-removing enzyme to make the product lactose-free).

I'm not a fan of switching to 'free-from' foods when we develop an intolerance, such as lactose or gluten, as it's an outward sign that all is not well with our internal microbiome. So if you feel better avoiding cow's milk, perhaps take a look at improving your gut health first (see Chapter 7), as this could well be a sign that something is amiss within. You could also try sheep or goat's milk instead, as these have smaller fat molecules, so many find they are more easily digested.

Plant 'milks'

I dislike the term 'plant milk'. In reality, they're 'plant waters' (mostly H_2O), with the addition of a few ingredients such as intensively cultivated oats, almonds or soya beans, plus some synthetic additives. They're only called 'milks' because they're white liquids and can be used in a similar way, but that's where the nutritional similarity ends. As you've probably gathered, I'm not a fan of processed plant milks, especially as these usually contain refined polyunsaturated seed oils (which, as we've seen, are more likely to cause inflammation in the body – see page 125) as well as synthetic vitamins and minerals that the body finds harder to absorb than those occurring naturally in animal milk. They can also have a huge carbon footprint when it comes to transportation. On the subject of sustainability, almond milk seems to be one of the worst offenders, as it takes a litre of water to grow a single almond – not very eco. Oat milk is popular as it froths up well in cappuccinos, but the downside here is that it is likely to be high in glyphosate pesticide residues and is one of the highest for spiking our blood glucose levels, as it contains twice as much carbohydrate as real milk.

Here are a few of the most popular milks and alternatives, with their most important metrics:

Type	Protein/ 100ml	Calcium/ 100ml	Glycaemic Index
Whole milk	3.5g	124mg	35–40
Semi-skimmed milk	3.6g	124mg	35–40
Skimmed milk	3.6g	130mg	35–40
Soya drink (Alpro organic)	3.3g	123mg *	50
Oat drink (Oatly)	1g	120mg *	60
Almond drink (Rude Health)	0.5g	120mg *	79–92
No Sugars Almond Drink (Rude Health)	0.6g	8mg	25
Coconut drink (Alpro original)	0.1g	120mg*	97

*artificially fortified

In terms of protein content, calcium supplies and a lower glycaemic index (reduced sugar spikes), real milk is the clear winner, not to mention being inexpensive and supportive of small-scale, family dairy farmers. If you're looking for a cheap and easy alternative though, my advice is to make your own oat 'milk' by simply soaking a handful of organic oats in water overnight and straining the liquid (adding a pinch of rock or sea salt for flavour). Oats do contain phytates, saponins and lectins, but these are reduced by soaking. This is by far the least expensive and most sustainable option, costing just a few pence and versatile for foaming into lattes, using on cereals or making smoothies. Do be aware that oat milk's anti-nutrient content may slightly lower the absorption of iron, zinc and calcium (see page 113), so factor this into your own nutritional needs. As for me, I'm sticking to buying real milk in glass bottles from my milkman or local dairy (good to see these delivery services expanding now) and am pleased to see the rise of refillable milk vending machines and wider availability of non-plastic packaging on the supermarket shelves, something to ask for if your supermarket doesn't already do. There's also a growing band of organic dairies offering organic, raw A2 milk and many now supply mail order too (have a look online), along with raw milk kefir and other probiotic dairy products. Milk freezes well, so you can consider bulk-buying for the freezer.

Yes please to cheese!

I love all kinds of cheese and look for cheeses made by smaller cheesemakers, rather than the more mass-market kind. Artisan cheeses tend to be made with grass-fed milk for better flavour, and are more likely to support smaller-scale, family-run farms. Goat and sheep cheeses are more easily digested, as their fat molecules are smaller, so may be better tolerated by those sensitive to dairy produce. I don't buy anything labelled as 'low-fat' and that goes for cheese too, especially as the fat content is where you'll find the flavour.

A Good Egg

I love an egg! Especially an organic one from a happy hen allowed to live free from caged confinement. If the government ever decides to appoint an egg Tsar, I'm their woman! Inexpensive, widely available, sustainable, versatile and tasty, just one egg contains a third of the recommended daily value of vitamin B7, plus small amounts of many of the other B vitamins. Nutritionally, eggs contain just about everything we need to live except for vitamin C. They're a cheap, easy and remarkably good source of protein, with nutritional scientists giving eggs an amino acid score of 100 and the highest net protein utilisation rate of all foods. In terms of protein composition, eggs have more sulphur-containing amino acids than other sources of protein, important for methylation which we'll come on to later (see page 291).

Eggs consist of four distinct parts: the egg white, yolk, membrane and shell, all of which have nutritional benefits. Egg whites are pure protein and have been shown to increase muscle mass and overall body strength, lower cholesterol levels and reduce visceral fat in the body (the kind of dangerously invisible fat that wraps itself around internal organs, even in those who appear very slender). Egg whites also contain cystine, a type of sulphur-containing amino acid shown to reduce serum cholesterol levels. This type of amino acid is also a precursor to glutathione (see page 66), so will have antioxidant properties too. Egg yolks contain phospholipids which suppress cholesterol absorption, with studies suggesting this also supports healthy bone growth. In the past, egg yolks have been wrongly linked with raising cholesterol, with repeated studies showing that, for most of us (unless suffering from a specific, hereditary disease such as familial hypercholesterolaemia, FH, which affects about 1 in 250 people), eating eggs has no effect whatsoever on our blood fats. This is because even if we eat lots of cholesterol, the body is clever enough to synthesise it in the liver, making it harmless.

In fact, the fats found in egg yolks actually *improve* healthy blood-fat ratios as well as boosting neurological health by feeding brain cells with important amounts of choline. The eggshells are also nutritious, being an excellent source of calcium that perhaps we should be grinding up and using instead of chucking onto the compost heap. When I kept my own chickens, I would pulverise the shells and feed them back to the hens to help strengthen their eggshells, but perhaps I should be adding them to my own shakes and smoothies? Even inside the shell, the membrane has been shown to have interesting properties, able to absorb toxins and heavy metals from the environment (it's used outside the food industry for this) and further studies show eggshell membrane to have anti-inflammatory effects, skin-moisturising properties and even the ability to specifically improve knee-joint pain, again possibly due to a high cysteine content. (By the way, those with joint pain could also consider supplementing with hyaluronic acid and collagen – see pages 295 and 292 – both helpful for lubricating connective tissues, as well as HRT, as oestrogen also eases joint soreness.)

In terms of ageing well, there can be few better, more easily available foods to help us along the way. Eating eggs has been shown to increase muscle strength, prevent sarcopenia (a gradual loss of muscle mass that occurs with ageing) and even speed muscle recovery in women over the age of 50, especially when combined with exercise (which I was especially pleased to discover, as I tend to follow my workouts at home with a couple of boiled eggs or an omelette). The precise number of eggs we should eat daily has not been established, with expert opinion ranging from one or two to as many as six daily. Personally, I hover around the two to three per day mark. I'll leave the last word with a meta-analysis on the benefits of eating eggs carried out by researchers at Kyushu University, Japan, published in the journal *Foods* in 2022, which concluded: 'Egg protein intake is expected to contribute to extending healthy life.'

A Fishy Issue

You'll have clocked that fish and seafood are all naturally high in both beneficial omega-3 fats and protein, so should we up our intake of fishy foods, especially when it comes to living well for longer? Fish and seafood are both very healthy food choices and, if bought from sustainable sources, they don't damage the delicate ocean environment either. Choose fish that are pole- or line-caught, not dredged from the ocean's fragile seabeds, and be picky with your species and avoid buying from depleted fish stocks. Here in the UK, most of our fish comes from 'the big five', namely cod, salmon, haddock, tuna and prawns, but being a maritime nation, over 150 different species of fish are caught in British waters. Cornish hake is a good option, as is handline-caught mackerel. Cornish sardines (the rebranded pilchard) is one of the fish highest in omega-3s and is now sustainably caught. Dover sole also scores well on the sustainability front, as do most shellfish.

When deciding which kinds of fish to eat, we also need to have a conversation around pollution. Concerns are rising over the increasing levels of 'forever chemicals', such as dioxins like polychlorinated biphenyls (dl-PCBs), accumulating in oily fish and seafood especially. One way to reduce our exposure is to remove the skin before cooking, as well as any fish fat (where toxins tend to accumulate), the 'tomalley' or soft green substance of lobster and 'mustard' or yellowish substance found inside crabs. White-fleshed fish, lower in fish fat/oil, are a better bet pollutant-wise, and watch out for deep-sea fish coming from overseas, such as swordfish and tuna, as these tend to be very high in mercury (as well as more often unsustainably fished).

Tuna contains mercury because they feed on smaller fish, already contaminated with mercury from industrial pollution and volcanic eruptions (as well as trillions of microplastic particles). These toxins are not easily excreted and so build up in the tissues of the tuna. Different types of tuna contain different levels of contamination – the least worst being light tuna (tinned) with around 10mcg mercury in an 85g portion, compared to Albacore tuna (fresh, frozen, jarred or tinned) at around 30mcg mercury per 85g. I personally don't often eat tuna for this reason and suggest it's not a regular part of any menu, especially for children and pregnant women. If I do eat it, I buy brands that state they are sustainably sourced and packed in olive oil – more expensive for sure, but it's not a staple on my shopping list.

Provided seafood is cultivated in clean waters, it will be relatively free of pollutants. Oysters, mussels, cockles and whelks used to be an everyday part of the British diet in the nineteenth century, but have fallen out of flavour favour. A pity, when they are nutritionally excellent and don't use any additional water supplies to farm. Even some vegans are OK with eating oysters as, like clams, mussels, whelks and cockles, they are headless invertebrates (with no spinal column) and are not sentient creatures, so don't feel pain (yet they are living organisms, which means technically they can't be considered a vegan food). The vast majority of oysters are farmed sustainably and oyster farming actively purifies the water they're grown in, capturing carbon along the way and making their farming a positive environmental activity. Nutritionally, oysters are an excellent source of complete protein and brain-healthy omega-3s, are especially rich in zinc and contain good amounts of iron, magnesium, selenium and vitamin B12. Ultimately, it's down to whether someone, vegan or not, appreciates their chewy texture and salty taste (and is comfortable with the philosophy alongside their high cost). Personally, I'm a fan and I love them as an occasional treat.

Another key nutrient found in fish and seafood is iodine, although this is less present in oily fish. You'll find good supplies in white fish such as haddock and cod (around 390mcg and 230mcg respectively). Yet again our friend the oyster scores highly here, with 144mcg iodine per 90g (half a dozen oysters), compared to a small tin of salmon (63mcg) or tuna (10mcg). Note: when it comes to iodine, cow's milk is also an excellent source (57mcg in a single large glass).

On a nutritional level, it's the oily kind of fish that gives us the highest levels of omega-3 essential fatty acids. An easy way to remember which ones are best is the mnemonic SMASH, which stands for:

- Sardines
- Mackerel
- Anchovies
- Salmon
- Herring

All are very good sources of brain-boosting fats, also more easily available in fish oil, krill and algae supplements, which I'll cover in more detail on page 227. Other excellent sources of iodine are seaweeds, highly sustainable as these sea veggies naturally grow in salt water, of which our planet has plenty, and are simply harvested by trimming by hand whereupon they simply regrow. I buy dried seaweed 'crisps' to snack on, usually made from sheets of nori, and also chop these up into small flakes to sprinkle over everything savoury from soups to salads (they're especially good with eggs too).

One of the most significant recent studies on human mortality (the American Million Veteran Program, 2022) found that a lower intake of animal foods (meat, eggs, fish and dairy) is associated with higher mortality. Over many years of researching what we eat and its effects on our physical and mental health, I've come to realise that our bodies are designed to eat a wide variety of naturally wholesome foods, not exclude them. I've become more aware of 'ancestral eating', that is eating in the way humans have evolved to eat over the millennia, and not influenced by the swift U-turns revolving around processed food and drink. It's clear that we need many vital nutrients from our food that are *only* naturally available, in the right ratios, in the animal kingdom – and that we lose these from our daily diets at our peril. These include nutrients needed for healthy brains, eyes, skin, muscles and bones. I'm talking about retinol (the exclusively animal form of vitamin A, which functions differently from the plant form beta-carotene), EPA, DHA and CLA fats found in fish and meat (see pages 105 and 116), heme iron, creatine, choline, taurine, vitamin D3, zinc . . . So yes, I do now eat unprocessed meat and dairy (and some line-caught fish or sustainably sourced seafood, such as Cornish crab), always with a watchful eye on how an animal has been reared and where it comes from.

Of course, some of these vital nutrients can be synthetically made and artificially added to fortify processed foods, but there is a problem here. The addition of synthetic vitamins back into looka-like foods, such as faux meat, simply doesn't work that well as they're not as well recognised and as fully absorbed by the body as those naturally occurring in real food. Do keep this in mind when reading labels on *any* processed food.

Fruit and Veg

We all know the importance of eating fruit and vegetables, from being told as children to 'eat your greens', 'an apple a day keeps the doctor away', 'carrots make you see in the dark', 'eat five-a-day', etc. Yet many of these messages are either not true or have little evidence to back them up. That's not to say that we shouldn't eat more veg, just that it's important to swallow some with a pinch of salt (both literally and metaphorically).

Perhaps the most pervasive message is the 'five-a-day' taken by almost all of us to be gospel truth. But, truth be told, it was a marketing exercise, invented in 1991 at a meeting of the fruit and veg companies in California, invested in by supermarket chains and since trademarked by the American National Cancer Institute. It is not actually supported by science and the studies funded to promote it produced mixed results, including one data set showing that the more fruit and vegetables eaten, the increased risks of cancer and shorter life expectancy. Around 3 billion kilos of pesticides are applied to fruit and vegetables each year globally, and there's every chance traces of these poisonous chemicals end up in our systems. Could eating more fruit and veg actually be contributing to our toxic overload, perhaps even triggering cancerous cell changes? It's a question worth considering. I'm not saying don't eat fruit and vegetables. What I am suggesting is that we should always question 'the science', especially when it's industry-funded. Eating organically grown fruit and veg wherever possible is one way to reduce pesticide exposure (see box on next page for tips on how to eat more organic food on a budget).

My advice for midlife and beyond is to limit the vegetables grown below the ground (especially potatoes, parsnips and carrots) as these are higher in carbohydrate (sugars) than others, especially the green, leafy kind. There are a few notable exceptions – I highly rate beetroot for its ability to improve our nitric oxide content, which increases blood flow and supports that all-important mitochondrial function (see page 62).

I'm also a big fan of anything from the brassica family, such as all kinds of cabbage, broccoli, rocket (arugula), cauliflower and Brussels sprouts, as not only do they contain high levels of vitamins (C, E and K as well as beta-carotene) and many minerals, they also uniquely contain glucosinolates, converted into isothiocyanates, shown to help fight cancer cells. These are especially concentrated in rocket and broccoli, two of my all-time favourites. I'm also a big fan of watercress, as this too contains a specific isothiocyanate, shown to be particularly protective against breast and lung cancer, switching 'off' certain cancer signals – among other cell-protective properties – but it must be eaten raw or very lightly cooked so as to preserve these unique properties. By contrast, I don't often each spinach or kale, as although these leafy greens are rich in vitamins, they are also high in oxalic acid, an anti-nutrient that interferes with our calcium absorption and can cause kidney and gallstones.

Eight ways to eat organic food on a budget

1. Eat less but better meat: cheap, intensively produced animal products are, in reality, more costly when you factor in health, animal welfare and environmental factors, often paid for down the line by the consumer in the form of additional taxes needed to clean up the waterways polluted by chemical run-off from intensive agriculture.

2. Grow your own: even a kitchen windowsill can provide cut-and-come-again salad leaves, cherry tomatoes and helpful herbs.

3. Subscribe to a fruit-and-veg box: there are plenty of options on the market nowadays.

4. Eat seasonally and from local suppliers, at least from UK producers and growers: we have some of the highest food-production standards in the world and the further fresh produce has to travel, the more likely it is to have been chemically 'preserved' in some way. This also helps reduce environmental transport and shipping costs.

5. Use your freezer: sift through the reduced section of supermarkets to find discounted organic food to pop in your freezer and stock up.

6. Look out for own-brand organic: this can further cut costs on your total food bill.

7. Make small swaps: just focusing on your staples to start with can still make a difference, according to experts.

8. Reduce food waste: make organic vegetable stocks from scraps of veggies or use bones from organic cuts of meat to whip up some bone broth. Avoid over-buying and try to use up the older items in your fridge in soups etc before restocking.

How to read food labels

Look for the following before you buy:

- Choose packaged foods with as few ingredients as possible.

- Watch out for ingredients that you don't recognise, such as emulsifiers and other food additives. Give anything with a long and complicated list of chemical additives a wide swerve. In the words of leading food writer Michael Pollan: 'don't eat anything your great-grandmother wouldn't recognise as food' – a very good rule to live by.

- Check provenance – does the label say precisely where the food comes from and not just where it was packed?

- When buying meat, has the animal been grass-fed or pasture-reared (or is there just a pretty picture of grass on the packaging)?

- Look for certified organic or at least free-range, especially when buying meats.

- The MSC (Marine Stewardship Council) is a good certification mark to look out for when buying fish, such as tuna.

Chocolate: Now for the Good News!

Chocolate is good for us. Yes, really. Not the highly processed junk chocolate filled with more sugar than anything else . . . no, I'm talking about the strong black stuff. Did you know that dark chocolate is actually the richest plant source of health-giving polyphenols? These plant chemicals protect our cells from inflammation, improve brain function and support our immune and cardiovascular health. It's positively medicinal . . . Chocolate (or, more specifically, cacao, the pod that's ground into powder) contains theobromine, similar to caffeine in that it gives us a lift, enhances mood and makes us feel more alert. Meta-analysis published in the *American Journal of Clinical Nutrition* shows chocolate and cacao to help improve heart health, lower blood pressure and improve insulin regulation, with researchers concluding, 'We found consistent acute and chronic benefits of chocolate or cocoa . . . with no suggestion of negative effects.'

As well as being a healthy, sweet snack, evidence is emerging that we should eat chocolate for pro-ageing and longevity too. Studies published in 2022 show that cacao assists apoptosis (the recycling of old cells), improves mitochondrial activity and rejuvenates senescent cells (see pages 55 and 62). Cacao has also been shown to help regulate gene expression, downregulating troublesome genetic 'snips' or variances (see page 49). One study even found it effective at reducing presbycusis, or age-related hearing loss (which currently has no effective treatment). Cacao also contains epicatechin, a compound linked to angiogenesis, the body's process of stem-cell regeneration. A study by researchers in California demonstrated that epicatechin-rich cocoa significantly increased capillary density (in mice, but, as we've seen, these studies are relevant to humans – see page 64) after just two weeks. This increase was due to a rise in stem-cell production, enabling tissues to repair themselves more quickly and effectively. So taking dark chocolate on hospital visits post-surgery is clinically a very good idea. Not just for repair work, though – the process of angiogenesis is critical throughout our lifespan, especially when it comes to ageing. By increasing blood-vessel growth, nutrients can be delivered more effectively around the body, and waste matter and toxic cell debris more easily removed. This, in turn, improves overall cell functioning, reduces inflammation and can help with pain management too.

Raw cacao beans also contain powerful antioxidant phenolic compounds (notably procyanidins) that reduce the oxidative stress that damages cells, leading to ageing and degenerative diseases, such as Alzheimer's. Cacao also stimulates endorphins, those happy chemicals in the brain which are also analgesic, so help lower pain and can even improve our quality of sleep (just don't eat dark chocolate close to bedtime as its caffeine content can keep you awake).

So, there's nothing intrinsically 'bad' about chocolate, it's more the extra ingredients we find in it that are troublesome. I buy plain cacao nibs and keep a stash of these in my kitchen for when I feel like grabbing something sweet – they're high in fibre and give us a healthy shot of antioxidants as well as satisfying a craving for something sweet. I eat a few of these plain, sprinkled into yoghurt or with a teaspoonful of nut butter for an instant Snickers bar-style bite. Of course, you can also choose a chocolate bar and, here, the key is to look for the percentage of cocoa solids it contains. The higher the percentage, the less room there is for added sugars and other ingredients, including fats such as palm oil.

I used to not like dark chocolate, having been brought up with the traditional milk chocolate bars and the kind of 'junk' bars we find in brightly coloured plastic wrappers to tempt us at the supermarket checkout or petrol station. However, it is possible to wean yourself off the sweeter stuff in stages. If you're a chocoholic who doesn't like dark varieties, try scaling up the percentage of cocoa each time you buy, gradually getting used to a slightly more bitter taste. I now find milk chocolate far too sweet and will always choose a darker option out of preference, buying some of the more niche brands that can be over 90 per cent cocoa, or even 100 per cent pure chocolate. A side benefit of these darker blends is that it's almost impossible to overeat, as one or two squares are all it takes to satisfy the sweetest tooth. Just keep in mind that all chocolate, especially the darker kinds, are high in caffeine. For this reason, I tend not to eat any after mid-afternoon and never after dinner.

Before buying any chocolate, it's worth checking the amount of sugar listed on the label. A simple switch can make a big difference in terms of reducing our sugar load. Alas, sugar levels in confectionery have sharply risen over the years, increasing on average by 23 per cent between 1992 and 2017. Check out the differences your choices make here:

Product	Sugar content per 100g
White chocolate	60g
Milk chocolate (average)	55g
Dark chocolate (70–85% cocoa)	22–26g
Keto dark chocolate (sweetened with stevia)	Less than 1g

What's the deal with heavy metals?

Set against all the good news and health benefits, a darker cloud has loomed large over some chocolate brands. Worrying studies surfaced in 2022 reporting traces of heavy metals, notably cadmium and lead, in dark chocolate, so how concerned should we be? Researchers from Consumer Reports, a US non-profit consumer organisation, measured heavy metals in 28 popular dark chocolate bars – and found cadmium and lead in all of them, including Godiva, Hershey's, Green & Black's, Lily's and Lindt. Even organic, ethical, vegan and sustainably sourced brands were not exempt from their findings. The only brands readily available in the UK found to contain below California's maximum acceptable dosage levels were Ghirardelli and Valrhona. Dark chocolate fared worse than milk chocolate simply because it has a higher content of pure cocoa solids. The National Confectioners Association said, 'the products cited in this study are in compliance with strict quality and safety requirements, and the levels provided to us by Consumer Reports testing are well under the limits established by our settlement.' Before ditching dark chocolate altogether, it's important to firstly remember that *all* plant foods tend to contain traces of heavy metals, depending on the soil they've been grown in. Chocolate is no exception. Cacao plants take up cadmium from the soil with the metal building up as the pod grows. Lead enters the food chain another way and seems to get into the cacao after the beans have been harvested, indicating it is more to do with the harvesting, drying and storage practices (and so is less linked to increased percentages in the cacao).

So do I still eat dark chocolate? Yes I do, especially for its pro-ageing and cell-protecting benefits, but I limit myself to just a few squares a day – and I check online for updated information from my favourite brands. Until we're clearer on the action taken by manufacturers to reduce heavy metals, I suggest this is the most prudent action for chocolate-lovers – enjoy modest amounts (although children and pregnant women should probably take extra care to limit their intake). Don't forget that cacao has been shown to be cellularly protective and we can also compensate by making sure our diets include other nutrients that protect us against heavy-metal harm, such as calcium, iron, selenium, glutathione, vitamin C and zinc.

My Day on a Plate

I mostly eat two meals a day: brunch and supper. This works for me and there is increasing evidence to support what's known as time-restricted eating (TRE), which I'll chat about in more detail in the next chapter. Here's what a typical day for me might look like:

Brunch (around 11am)

My first mouthful is always a quality protein with some healthy fats. Boiled eggs, an omelette, scrambled eggs or some avocado on a bed of broccoli drizzled with a bit of olive oil are just a few of my favourites. I also love a nice bowl of thick, plain, live yoghurt (Greek is great), topped with nuts and seeds for added crunch and a sprinkling of blueberries, raspberries or chopped apple. If I'm still hungry, or fancy a snack a bit later, I'll toast a piece of sourdough, smother this with butter and/or olive oil and add a few slices of cheese (I love Gruyere and Manchego for their strong, nutty flavour and higher calcium content), avocado or almond butter. This keeps me feeling full until supper time. When I have no time to prep anything, I'll throw together a protein shake or pop some overnight organic oats in a jar with yoghurt, grated apple and berries and take this with me on my travels.

Supper (around 7pm)

I'll always plan this around what my protein is going to be – perhaps some simply cooked chicken, fish, red meat or seafood; maybe a cheese toastie or even a soufflé (easier to make than you might think!); or some tofu or grilled halloumi. Next come the veggies – always something green, such as broccoli, cabbage, leeks, green beans, edamame beans or peas, with the occasional artichoke or asparagus, if in season, as a gut-friendly treat. I use quite a few different seasonings and spices to add plant diversity to my meals, and always have red onions, garlic, ginger and turmeric on hand, together with fresh herbs grown in pots on my kitchen windowsill (parsley, basil, chives, mint and oregano are some of my favourites).

Eating protein and healthy fats first means I rarely get sugar cravings now, but if I do fancy something sweet after supper, I'll go for a handful of cashews or almonds, yoghurt with ground almonds and seasonal fruit (the summer is great for fresh peaches, greengages and plums), a fresh orange or a couple of satsumas.

I live by the 80:20 rule when it comes to my meals: eating as above 80 per cent of the time, with 20 per cent of my meals being more relaxed and available for 'treats', such as eating out or celebration cakes. However, the older I have become, the more I have learnt that these are not 'treats' but 'threats' to the way I look and feel – and over time they have become far less attractive.

My snacks

These are the things I keep in my fridge or cupboard and always like to have on hand, either for snacking or to throw together a quick 'snack plate' supper. Stock up with these and clear out the c**p. If it's not in the house, you can't eat it.

- Brazil nuts: a great source of selenium; I eat two a day
- Almonds: all kinds – whole, flaked and ground
- Walnuts: good for snacking on or sprinkling over salads, yoghurt, or whatever!
- Peanuts in their shells: if I get the munchies (usually while watching a movie or a boxset), I'll grab a bag of monkey nuts. It's impossible to eat these quickly and the action of cracking them open (or any other kind of nut, such as pistachios which

have the highest melatonin content of any food, so a great late-night snack!) slows the process and prevents overeating

- Apples, satsumas, berries of all kinds, grapes
- Stone fruit, such as plums, peaches and apricots (less sugar than tropical fruits)
- Under-ripe bananas: these contain less sugar; just chew thoroughly as they are harder to digest
- Greek yoghurt
- Kefir
- High-protein, thin bagels: I keep these pre-sliced in the freezer ready to toast and smother in olive oil and nut butter if I get a carb craving
- Slices of cheese (not the fake, processed kind, check the label)
- Hummus
- Carrot sticks soaking in brine: a delicious salty snack
- Olives: all kinds!
- Fennel, celery, cucumber, red pepper, baby courgettes and chicory: all good for crunching on
- Taramasalata
- Soya beans: either in the pod (edamame-style) or I buy bags of frozen soya beans and keep a dish of salted beans in the fridge, ready to dip into
- Protein shakes: I mostly use a casein protein or unflavoured bone broth powder (see page 137) and whizz this up with a glass of milk, adding half a banana, yoghurt, kefir, ground almonds and/or a handful of berries if I'm really hungry

Kitchen cupboard staples
It's helpful to have a range of healthy foods, flavourings and condiments to cheer up simple protein dishes. These are the things you'll always find in my kitchen:

- Apple cider vinegar (see page 182)
- Eggs: always organic and from pastured hens, if possible
- Organic short-grain brown rice: I buy this in bulk online as I love its nutty flavour and the whole family love it too
- Frozen peas, broad beans and edamame beans
- HP sauce, just because I love the flavour of tamarind and it goes so well with eggs
- Balsamic vinegar glaze (just brilliant on mozzarella with a few pumpkin seeds – a meal in itself)
- Dijon and wholegrain mustard
- Fresh garlic and ginger root
- Sunflower and pumpkin seeds
- Turmeric, rock salt, black pepper, smoked paprika and home-grown dried herbs, including mint, bay leaves, rosemary and oregano

And these are the things you will always find in my fridge . . .

- Whole milk, plain live yoghurt and kefir
- Brassicas: cabbage, cauliflower, broccoli and the like, depending on the season
- Watercress
- A jar of anchovies and some chillies for seasoning
- Cheese: usually Parmesan or similar for grating, goat Gouda or Manchego (made from sheep's milk) for slicing, and some mozzarella balls (my kids' favourite!)
- Fresh basil and parsley, unless growing in a windowsill pot
- Blueberries: the *ultimate* berry

When it comes to looking at what we eat in order to age well and give our bodies the best chance for a healthier older age, it's important we reframe our view of fats, adding in more of the healthier kind and far fewer of those that damage our cells, as well as increasing the amount of protein we eat with each and every meal.

It's important to cook from scratch when we can, using wholesome, fresh, seasonal ingredients and really cutting back on the amount of foods we eat that have been processed or premade. Simplifying meals not only costs less, but liberates us from UPF addictions.

Healthy hacks

- Use butter, ghee, coconut oil or lard, never margarine or spread. And try not to eat anything fried, unless you've cooked it yourself in a healthy oil.
- Build meals around protein. Prioritise protein on your plate first, then add your veggies and healthy trimmings such as salads, pickles, fresh herbs and healthy oils.
- Avoid premade meals out of a packet as much as possible and try to steer clear of anything that isn't actually real food on the ingredients listing.

CHAPTER 5

Maintaining a Healthy Weight in Midlife

When it comes to weight loss, I prefer to think in terms of health gain with lost pounds as a beneficial side effect. Being 'overfat', to use the term used to describe the amount of visceral (hidden) fat around our internal organs, is the most important metric when it comes to weight loss. This is why measuring our weight against a conventional BMI table is so unreliable. BMI is calculated by dividing our weight in kilograms by our height in metres squared. The downside of doing this is that it misses a huge proportion of those of us with undiagnosed metabolic disease. Although BMI tables are widely used by GPs and dieticians, they are limited in usefulness and often wildly inaccurate due to the varying weight of the skeleton, water retention, ratio of fat versus muscle (muscle weighs more than fat, so you might be heavier, but leaner), as well as differences due to sex, age and race. This is why a professional UK wrestler (more muscle) has a similar BMI to a Japanese sumo wrestler (more fat), but very different health outcomes.

A more insightful measurement is your waist-to-height ratio. Simply divide your waist circumference (measured at the navel) by your height. Anything greater than 0.5 is a pretty good sign that you have excess body fat. For example, my height is 165cm and my waist measurement is 80cm (just under half my height, which would be 82.5cm, so I am doing OK). It's generally accepted that a healthy waist measurement is no more than 80cm for women. Excess unhealthy body fat – anything 0.5 or higher – increases the risk of heart disease, type 2 diabetes and breast cancer, with anything above 0.6 or higher being especially concerning (charts showing the danger zones are easily found online – just search 'height-to-waist ratio chart'). Carrying extra weight around our middles is an indication of excess fat building up around organs such as the liver and pancreas, which can cause insulin resistance as the insulin can't get through the fat. This means the insulin we produce can't work as it should, increasing the risk of having high blood glucose (sugar).

> **How insulin works**
> Insulin is a hormone produced by the pancreas when sugar enters the bloodstream. It enables the cells to produce energy from sugars when our glucose levels go up and also signals to the liver to store blood sugar. This, in turn, keeps our blood-glucose levels in check, as the liver then releases small amounts of glucose between meals.

Most diets don't work because they're boring and reek of deprivation; not a good mindset when it comes to how we approach one of life's great pleasures – eating! Dieting *per se* has proven to be pointless. An exhaustive study by the National Health and Nutrition Examination Survey published in 2019 revealed that 95 per cent of those who lose weight on a diet regain it within five years. Over the years, I've tried most diets – the egg 'n' grapefruit Scarsdale sensation of the eighties, macrobiotic, keto, paleo . . . I even joined WeightWatchers back in the nineties, which although useful for shifting a few pounds, didn't work for me in the long term. I'm also against any kind of slimming club that regards high-sugar snacks as 'sinful treats'. Sugar is not a 'treat' and framing sugary snacks as being a reward for 'good' behaviour misses the point of developing long-term and sustainable healthy eating habits.

Put your body first and fuel it with the best foods for it to function effectively and well.

So what actually works when it comes to long-term weight loss? The best 'diet' isn't a diet at all – it's a healthier way of eating. Ask yourself this question before you swallow *anything*: is this forkful going to have a positive or negative impact? Don't be obsessive, just follow the 80:20 rule of eating (and drinking) mostly good things, most of the time, and you won't go far wrong (see page 13).

In my experience, long-term weight loss comes down to the slow and steady dialling down of the pounds. Just as the extra weight we might be carrying around does not appear overnight, so any shedding of it will take some time too. If your weight has unhealthily crept up over many years, it's more realistic to expect many years to lose it too. Crash diets are exactly that – a crash of the body's metabolism and all the negative side effects that go with yo-yo dieting, when your metabolism gets so disrupted it no longer functions to burn energy from food in the most efficient way.

Understanding Your 'Set Point'

One of the reasons why the overwhelming majority of us who lose a large amount of weight will regain it is that each of us has our own individual 'set point' that governs how much our bodies weigh. This is a unique internal metric, based on genetics, how we live and our environments. Our set point is controlled by a part of the brain called the hypothalamus, located at the base of the brain, which controls (among other things) body temperature and how much fat we need to conserve in order to function. Once we dip below our optimum weight, or set point, our hypothalamus switches off the mechanisms for losing weight, so we plateau – no matter how well we restrict what's on our plates or how much vigorous exercise we do.

For those who've been overweight for a long time, it can be very hard to get the hypothalamus to readjust to a lighter reading on the scales, which is why any weight gain is best shifted before it gets a grip. That's not to say it's impossible for someone who is very obese to return to a healthy weight, just that it will take more time and needs to be done slowly, consciously, with the realisation and acceptance that the body is unlikely to ever become a certain weight if that is not your body's natural genetic type. So please be kind to yourself. Small steps, taken slowly over time, really do lead to the best outcome in the long run.

Why Counting Calories Doesn't Work

Most of us grew up in an era when calorie counting seemed the obvious way to reduce weight, but the problem is that not all calories are created equal. How our bodies burn calories depends on many factors, including the type of food we're eating, our metabolism and even our gut microbes. Two people can eat exactly the same number of calories and yet the outcome can be very different when it comes to weight loss. When you think about it, counting calories doesn't actually make much sense: two hard-boiled eggs contain about the same number of calories as a small 45g bag of Skittles (around 180kcal), but the fats and protein in the eggs will keep us feeling fuller for longer (the satiety factor), whereas scoffing a few handfuls of sugary sweets just sends our blood sugars soaring – leaving us feeling even hungrier than before, so we eat even more. The calories that come from UPFs have also been shown to cause the greatest weight gain when compared to exactly the same number of calories that come from natural, whole foods cooked from scratch. So, trust me on this: stop counting calories! If you want something to count, count the grams of sugars you're eating. I switch to eating only naturally low-sugar foods (or those sweetened with sugar-free alternatives such as stevia or monk fruit – see page 180) containing less than 5g sugars per 100g if I'm trying to shift a few pounds.

Just as we don't need to count calories, we should also stop obsessing over our food. Hypervigilance over every mouthful is not only unnecessary, but can also lead to disordered eating and orthorexia (an unhealthy obsession with 'healthy' eating – of any kind). I'm more in favour of 'intuitive eating', a personalised approach based on internal cues, with a genuine focus on wellbeing (as in feeling really well) not weight loss, which automatically follows as a beneficial side effect. My view is that if the body is functioning well, running on the foods it actually needs for energy, mental health and physical strength, the excess pounds are far more likely to be shed. It may take a bit more time, but it will avoid the ups and downs of the more depressing diets and – more importantly – free up our moods and minds to focus on more life-enhancing things.

> **Go low-carb**
>
> This doesn't mean cutting out carbs completely, but swapping out refined carbs (white flour, potatoes, white rice and sugars) for the more complex kind. Refined carbohydrates contain one type of sugar which the body breaks down very quickly, causing blood sugars to rise. Complex carbohydrates, by contrast, as we've seen (page 131), contain three or more sugars joined together, resulting in a more gradual energy release which the body is better able to cope with without causing sudden blood-sugar 'spikes'. Examples of complex carbs include sweet potatoes, leafy greens and other non-starchy veggies, nuts, seeds and whole grains, such as brown rice, beans and pulses. This might be a bowl of wholewheat (brown) pasta, chili con carne made with kidney beans or wholemeal tortillas.

Time-Restricted Eating for Weight Loss

Another fascinating area of weight-loss and health-gain research is time-restricted eating (TRE), a form of intermittent fasting. Studies show that eating within a 10–12-hour window (or shorter) improves our blood-sugar response, actively supports the good gut bacteria involved with metabolism and helps with weight loss. This is especially helpful for those with type 2 diabetes or who have been diagnosed as being pre-diabetic. Sounds hard to do? In reality, it's very simple.

The best time length for TRE is to find an 'eating window' that you personally find easy to adopt and stick to (we're all different here!). You may find giving up breakfast to be the easiest option or you may simply not be able to function without that early-morning energy boost. When I first tried getting up and on with my day without breakfast, I will admit I found it hard. We've been so programmed in our psyche to get up and grab a bowl of cereal, or at least a piece of toast or sugary snack, but I soon realised that it was more a matter of psychologically getting over the mental panic of skipping breakfast. Once I rationalised that, actually, I wasn't starving hungry, I'd eaten well the night before, spent the night asleep and could go a few more hours before my first mouthful, the process was surprisingly easy. It literally took just two or three days of me telling myself that I was going to be fine – and that food was, indeed, on its way – for my 'hunger brain' to calm down. I generally have my first bite of brunch at around 11am, sometimes even later. In practice, this means that I mostly eat two meals a day: brunch and supper (see page 164 for my day on a plate). And by choosing to eat high-fat, high-protein foods first thing, I've also smoothed out my energy slumps and no longer crave a bit of cake or reach for the biscuit tin at teatime.

You may find the opposite 'eating window' works better for you. Maybe you've tried skipping breakfast only to find yourself on the floor with zero energy come mid-morning. In that case, fuel up first thing, have lunch and bring your evening meal forward to much earlier in the day. The science suggests that it doesn't make a whole heap of difference which way round you approach your food gap – just make sure there is one! Studies have been digging into the various different 'eating windows' to try to find the best length of gap to give the digestive system a break. The most successful eating window – in terms of results and actual adherence for those on measured trials – has been found to be 10–12 hours of eating, followed by a 14–12-hour break.

Use this at-a-glance chart for easy calculations and highlight what works best for you:

Fasted time	Last mouthful (finish supper)	First mouthful (first food)
14 hours	6pm	8am
	7pm	9am
	8pm	10am
	9pm	11am
	10pm	12 noon
12 hours	6pm	6am
	7pm	7am
	8pm	8am
	9pm	9am
	10pm	10am
10 hours	6pm	4am
	7pm	5am
	8pm	6am
	9pm	7am
	10pm	8am

While fasting, you can drink water, black tea or coffee or herb teas. Some experts say that sugar-free flavourings, such as stevia, are OK to have while in a fasted state, but others point to research showing that the body produces an insulin response to anything sweet (even if zero calorie, due to their sweet taste confusing the pancreas), so I tend to avoid any flavourings.

Why Sugar Should be Avoided

We've already seen how *all* forms of carbohydrates convert into sugars once we eat them, but what about the pure, white stuff itself? Sugar is a non-nutrient, meaning that it doesn't provide any nutritional value whatsoever. We just don't need it – plain and simple – but especially when it comes to weight loss.

According to the NHS, adults should eat less than 30 grams of 'free sugars' a day. In practical terms, the UK recommended sugar intake is no more than 7–8 teaspoons a day for men and 5–6 teaspoons for women. This is a maximum recommended limit – not a daily target! Free sugars are exactly that – not those bound up in the cells of the food we eat. Free sugars are added to food or drinks and include sugars found naturally in honey, syrups and fruit juices. Better choices are 'intrinsic sugars', those naturally found in foods, slowed by fibre, fats and other nutrients, such as milk or natural yoghurt and fresh or dried fruit (small amounts as their sugars are highly concentrated) and vegetables. A study published in the *British Medical Journal* (*BMJ*) found that almost all cakes and biscuits sold in the UK contain more than 22.5g of sugar per 100g. This means that just one biscuit can take us close to the NHS recommended limit of 30g daily. Just ONE biscuit.

As we all know, sugar is everywhere, added to just about every processed food, even savoury ones. A 2007 survey by *Which?* magazine found that Asda's sticky chilli chicken and Tesco's crispy beef with sweet chilli sauce contained more sugar per gram than vanilla ice cream. There are more than 50 different names for sugar, and the food industry continues to find new and inventive words for hiding it in plain sight (see list on the next page). To further 'hide' the sugar content of foods, manufacturers split the amount of it listed on labels into separate ingredients, such as corn syrup, maltose, dextrose and so on. Any food ingredient needs to appear in order of greatness on a label so we can see what we're eating most of. By listing many different forms of sugars as sub-ingredients, they are moved further down the list, making them less obvious and harder to spot.

Powerful lobbies fight hard to avoid front-of-packet labelling and it can be difficult to figure out exactly how much of the white stuff we're stuffing. The key is to know that 1 teaspoon = just over 4 grams of sugar. So if a food label says a portion (say 100g) contains 25g of sugars (listed under 'carbohydrate' on the label), that means it contains a little over 6 teaspoons of sugar.

Watch out for the words 'serving size' as this often underplays how much we might actually have as a portion.

Here's how to spot sugar in its most common guises:

- Agave
- Beet sugar or concentrate
- Blackstrap molasses
- Coconut or palm sugar
- Corn syrup (especially high-fructose corn syrup), or any 'syrup'
- Fruit juice concentrate
- Fruit purée
- Glucose, fructose, maltose, sucrose, lactose, dextrose . . . (basically anything ending in 'ose')
- Grape concentrate
- Honey

- Invert sugar
- Maple syrup

If you're looking to lose weight, as well as protect metabolic health as you age, choose foods with no more than 5g per 100g listed on the ingredient label. This is harder than it sounds – check it out! – but worth it if you want to wean yourself off the white stuff. This is the general rule I live by, with exceptions for a conscious decision to eat something sweet. Coming back to the 80:20 rule again (see page 13).

Sugar substitutes

So what about sugar substitutes? Should we simply switch to an artificial sweetener for our sugar fix? The answer here is mixed, as it depends on which substance we're talking about, but it's worth noting that an exhaustive 2019 review of over 50 studies on non-sugar sweeteners (NSS) in 2018 found *no* difference in weight loss when used. In fact, a study by the University of Texas Health Science Center at San Antonio showed that, rather than promoting weight loss, the use of diet drinks was a marker for increasing weight gain and obesity. Those who consumed diet soda were more likely to gain weight than those who consumed naturally sweetened soda – and animal studies have convincingly proven that artificial sweeteners cause body weight gain. How can this be the case if they have no calories? Obviously, all artificial sweeteners have a sweet taste and this causes an insulin response, causing blood sugar to rise which may then be stored as fat. In the Texan experiment, rats given artificial sweetener steadily increased their caloric intake, increasing their body weight, making them fatter . . .

So it would seem that there are few real benefits of artificial sweeteners and some, such as acesulfame K/potassium (E950), aspartame (E951), erythritol (E968), saccharin (E954), sorbitol (E420) and sucralose (E955), have been linked to health risks ranging from neurological disorders, heart disease, cancer and hormone disruption to behavioural and cognitive problems, headaches, anxiety, depression, insomnia and gastrointestinal symptoms. And for some of the newer ones on the market, little is known about their longer-term health effects, especially their impact on our gut health. Ultimately, it's up to you whether you choose to use sugar substitutes. My advice would be to avoid them altogether if you can and instead use small amounts of natural sugars in your daily food and drinks if you really need to – with a few notable exceptions, listed below.

Monk fruit

Extracted from luo han guo or 'Buddha fruit', it's 100–250 times sweeter than sugar. Relatively new to the market, there are few reports of adverse effects and its natural antioxidants may even have helpful anti-inflammatory properties. Studies (in mice) have shown that it can actually help reduce blood-sugar levels and it would appear to be a potentially good alternative to using sugar.

Stevia/stevioside/steviol glycosides (E960)

Made from the leaves of the stevia plant, it's 100–300 times sweeter than sugar. Some find it slightly bitter in taste, but the newer (more expensive) forms of water extraction seem to overcome this. Studies have shown that it may help lower insulin and glucose levels. You'll find it in health food shops as it is considered a safe, natural alternative to sugar. You can even grow your own plant and use the leaves in teas and cooking at home.

Xylitol (E967)

A natural substance with a similar level of sweetness to sugar, xylitol is found in fruits and vegetables, and is often used in chewing gums and minty sweets. Aside from being a sweetener, xylitol's main claim to fame is its benefits for teeth as it raises the pH in the mouth, preventing the growth of bacteria that cause cavities. It withstands cooking and can be used in baking, but large amounts will have a laxative effect. (NB: all sweeteners from the polyols family (such as sorbitol and erythritol) can have a laxative effect if eaten in large quantities.) Xylitol is highly toxic for dogs.

How to reduce sugar cravings
- Start the day with protein and healthy fats, so as not to trigger an insulin spike which can make you crave more sugar.
- Getting better sleep has been shown to reduce cravings.
- Eating more slowly helps.
- Choose high-protein, low-carb snacks, such as boiled eggs, cheese and also nuts (to a lesser extent).
- Swap milk chocolate for dark.

Supplements to Support Weight Loss

When it comes to effective weight loss, there's no replacement for the golden rule of eating more healthy fats and protein with fewer sugars, but there are a few supplements that can be a useful support act. These are the ones I rate:

Apple cider vinegar

Not strictly speaking a supplement, but it can be used as a healthy weight-loss habit, which can reduce a glucose spike by around one third, thanks to the action of the acetic acid on the digestive system. It works by slowing down the rate glucose is released from food, giving our muscles time to soak up the extra glucose as it enters the bloodstream. This then reduces the chance of sudden sugar spikes overloading the body and getting stored as fat. Any kind of vinegar works for this (lemon juice is also effective), but the real stuff is made from crushed apples and water that have been allowed to naturally ferment over time, resulting in a cloudy liquid and a 'mother' of the apple (a gelatinous layer produced by the acetic acid bacteria that ferments the vinegar), which has the additional advantage of supporting our good gut bugs too (see more on page 209).

Dose: 1tbsp in water 20 minutes or so before meals (especially when eating carbs)

L-ornithine

This is a natural amino acid with many important roles in the body including those for liver and brain function. It can also help target fat around the middle and has been shown to stimulate the release of growth hormone, helping the body to convert fat into lean muscle. Animal studies showed significant abdominal fat reduction after nine weeks of supplementation. L-ornithine is a fussy supplement though and needs to be taken on a completely empty stomach (2.5 hours after your last mouthful), ideally at bedtime as it works with the body's natural hormone and circadian rhythms. Taking this on an empty stomach 20–30 minutes before a bit of high-intensity exercise (some squats or similar, so long as these make you breathless) can also activate its effects. Once taken, wait 1.5 hours before eating again.

Dose: 2,500mg daily

Spermidine

Spermidine is found in many foods (such as wheatgerm, soya beans and nuts) and the supplement form is often extracted from buckwheat (a gluten-free seed, despite its name). It has been shown to be helpful for supporting metabolic issues, with studies showing it can induce autophagy (as we saw in Chapter 2 – see page 57), reducing overall fat levels and improving insulin resistance. Spermidine also helps the digestive system make beneficial changes to our gut health and microbiomes, specifically those that are helpful for the metabolism of fats.

Dose: 800mg daily

Green tea

Unlike the so-called 'slimming tea' scam, green tea for weight loss is backed by science. It contains the antioxidant catechin EGCG, which can help rev up our metabolisms and break down fat cells by boosting the effects of the fat-burning hormone norepinephrine (noradrenaline). EGCG helps protect this hormone, enabling more fat to be broken down within the body. In particular, it seems to be especially beneficial for breaking down the visceral 'belly' fat around our middles. Drinking green tea delivers high levels of beneficial antioxidant catechins, but for fat loss, higher-strength supplements seem to be more effective. It also contains caffeine, so avoid drinking it at bedtime.

Dose: 300–600mg daily

Berberine

One of the newest buzzes for weight loss, berberine is a bright yellow extract that comes from plants such as barberry, Oregon grape and golden seal. Traditionally used as a natural antibiotic (it can help get rid of *H. pylori* infection – a common cause of peptic ulcers), the latest excitement here is around lowering blood sugar, cholesterol regulation and improved metabolic health. Clinical studies published in 2023 show berberine to be as effective as metformin (a common type 2 diabetes drug) for lowering glucose levels. These studies also showed a reduction in the waist measurements of women who took it, compared to the placebo. This has led to berberine being hailed as 'nature's Ozempic', the diabetes drug being privately prescribed for weight loss.

Dose: 500–1,000mg daily

Bergamot

Various brands of supplements use bergamot polyphenol fraction (BPF), extracted from bergamot, a bitter Italian citrus fruit, clinically proven to improve heart health and metabolism, as well as encouraging unhealthy fats to pass through the gut, also assisting cholesterol balance. These bergamot extracts work by improving the way fats are processed in the liver, in turn improving sugar balance and helping fatty liver issues.

Dose: 1,000mg daily

Glucomannan

This is a dietary fibre from the root of the konjac plant, also known as the elephant yam, which works by absorbing water in the stomach and intestines exceptionally well so that it swells and forms a bulky, fibrous gel. It works very simply, by taking up space in the stomach to create a feeling of fullness without actually eating any food. Useful for treating constipation, glucomannan is also helpful for gut health as it feeds our friendly bacteria, encouraging them to produce butyrate, shown to protect against fat gain. Glucomannan is available as a powder which you stir into a glass of water and drink quickly, before it forms its thick gel. It is also the main ingredient in shirataki 'diet', low-carb, virtually calorie-free rice and noodles, which work in the same way once cooked and eaten.

As with all food supplements, don't exceed the recommended daily dose on the pack as brand strengths do vary, and consult your doctor for any medication contraindications or personal medical concerns.

When it comes to weight loss, see food as a friend, not a foe. Do eat healthy fats and protein, but try to ditch the sugars. Don't obsess over calorie counting, but do count grams of sugars and avoid processed foods as much as possible, which are often deliberately designed to make us overeat. Your first meal of the day is the most important one – start how you mean to go on and get ahead by focusing on healthy fats and protein. This is the best way to avoid carb cravings later in the day and will keep you feeling fuller for longer. Never eat carbs on their own; get some fibrous veggies in the system first to slow down their glucose release. Consider extending the gap between your last mouthful of food in the evening and the first one of the day. Give your body an occasional break from food and avoid continual snacking. Taking a short walk after every meal also helps with fat loss.

Healthy hacks

- Fill your fridge and cupboards with sustaining snacks that will keep you away from biscuits, cakes and other sweet saboteurs. My favourites are Brazil nuts, olives, cheese, crunchy veggie sticks (cucumber, carrots, celery, red peppers, fennel . . .), hummus, taramasalata, plain live yoghurt and no-sugar oat cakes.
- Don't mistake thirst for hunger. If you feel hungry, have a large glass of water first – you'll often find that hunger pang melts away.
- Get in the habit of reading food labels, especially when it comes to sugar levels. Aim for foods containing fewer than 5g per 100g of sugars.
- Choose alternative sugar sweeteners carefully. My preferred options are monk fruit and stevia.

CHAPTER 6

You Are What You Drink

When deciding the best drinking habits to add to our health stacks, the starting place has to be water as the ultimate thirst-quenching refreshment. Staying hydrated is often overlooked when we talk about diet, but drinking enough water is crucial not only for health, but also for controlling blood-sugar levels. A lack of fluid in our bodies means there is a higher concentration of sugars in the blood, so the simple act of drinking more water lowers blood sugar. Just be careful not to overdo the fruit juices, which are very high in sugars (even the natural kind) as well as fizzy drinks, including so-called 'energy drinks'. I stick to a maximum of one small glass of fresh (not out of a bottle) juice a day, ideally diluted with water and sipped slowly. Juices, especially fruit, are packed with sugar and are more like energy-sappers as they surge blood sugars, leading to an exhausted slump. Plain water is good and I filter my tap water either with a simple jug filter or a built-in under-counter water filter. Make plain water a bit more interesting by adding a slice of lemon, cucumber or herbs – basil leaf water made with a spritz of lemon or lime is especially delicious. Sparkling water also helps ring the changes and feels a bit more of a 'drink'. But be wary of drinking too much plain water on its own, as this can lower your important electrolyte balance.

Water works

For a rough guide to optimum water intake, take your body weight in pounds, divide it in half, and that's the number of fluid ounces you should be drinking in a day. Little and often is the best option, so when you know how many fluid ounces you should be drinking for optimum hydration, divide this by the number of hours you're awake and try to drink this amount every hour. Drinking smaller amounts more frequently throughout the day has been shown to be up to 40 per cent more hydrating than glugging back a few large glasses because you suddenly remembered your water intake. How to tell at a glance if you're properly hydrated? Check your wee! It should be a pale straw colour – darker urine means you're likely to be dehydrated. If you're not used to drinking more water, increase your intake gradually and your kidneys will adjust to the additional volume and you'll need to 'go' less often.

How Electrolytes Support Our Health

Electrolytes are particles that carry a positive or negative electrical charge and, in nutritional terms, they're the essential minerals found in blood, sweat and urine. When these minerals are dissolved, such as in a glass of water, they form electrolytes that the body can use for all kinds of metabolic processes. The key ones include sodium (salt), potassium, calcium, magnesium and phosphate. As calcium and phosphate are common minerals in the diet, electrolyte drinks tend to focus on replenishing sodium, potassium and magnesium. These electrolytes, especially sodium, help us maintain the best fluid balance and correct blood pH levels within the body – crucial for energy and overall cell health.

The morning is an especially good time to replace our electrolytes as we dehydrate as we sleep, especially if the bedroom is centrally heated/too warm and/or we've had a hot night (be it a night of passion or hot flushes), or if we've drunk any alcohol the night before. I also have a glassful when I could do with some extra brain power to focus or concentrate on a project. Low levels of electrolytes leads to many symptoms, including tiredness, irregular heartbeat, confusion and headaches. If any of these sound familiar, replacing your electrolytes can have an immediate and profound effect on how you feel. Drinking an electrolyte drink is also more hydrating and reviving than plain water alone, as water dilutes our internal mineral balance without replenishing it.

It's especially helpful to replace electrolytes before drinking coffee as our caffeine-filled cuppa is diuretic, so lowers our sodium levels and reduces our overall hydration. Each cup of coffee depletes around 600mg sodium. Interestingly, black tea contains a little sodium, manganese, potassium and magnesium, so is not such an issue. Sodium intake should generally be around 3,000–5,000mg (1–1.5tsp) daily, but it's highly variable. You'll need more if you exercise and sweat more, or if you're perspiring when the weather's hot. Body weight is also a key factor for salt requirements – the bigger you are, the more you'll need.

Electrolyte drinks are especially beneficial before and after exercise too. In fact, studies show that we work out harder and for longer when fuelled by a better electrolyte balance. I like to make my own electrolyte drink (see recipe below) – an excellent wake-up refresher first thing (and no, this doesn't seem to adversely affect our fasted state – see page 174).

How to make electrolyte water

1 medium-sized glass of water (preferably filtered)

¼ teaspoon rock or sea salt (provides sodium)

Squeeze of fresh lemon or lime (provides potassium and vitamins C and B6)

Simply mix the ingredients together and stir with a teaspoon. I prep this the night before and keep it in my bathroom, ready to drink each morning after brushing my teeth. This mixture does not affect fasting or keto, but premade electrolyte drinks or powders may do if they contain any form of sugars/flavours.

NB As a shortcut, simply add a pinch of sea salt to a glass of water and stir to dissolve.

If you want to go one step even better, use a rock salt such as pink Himalayan, as this contains traces of useful micro-minerals too. Sea salt is also a good option as it contains trace minerals, although there have been concerns raised about micro-plastic particles in the ocean ending up in the salt shaker, including the plastic polymers polyethylene and polypropylene. Studies say the health risk is negligible at the moment, but this is something to keep an eye on. As for table salt, this contains the same amount of sodium as sea or rock salt, without the trace minerals. If you are using table salt, try to buy the iodised kind, as this is helpfully fortified with iodine.

I also buy zero-sugar electrolyte drinks and you'll find an increasing selection online, mostly sweetened with stevia, the herbal no-sugar flavouring we explored on page 181. My favourite brands include Body Bio, LMNT and Ancient And Brave, all easily mixed with water. LMNT has also generously shared how to make their original unflavoured electrolyte base at home – here's how:

½ teaspoon salt (provides ~1g sodium)
500mg potassium citrate powder (provides ~200mg potassium)
¼ teaspoon magnesium malate powder (provides ~60mg magnesium)

Mix together with anything from 500ml to 1 litre water, depending on how salty you like your drink!

Other Drinks Are Available . . .

Coffee, tea – and even wine – are, for many of us, everyday beverages, but are they good or bad? The answers may surprise you. Let's start with coffee.

The case for more coffee

I know many who have given up drinking coffee over the years, thinking this would be better for their health. Having researched its benefits, I've actually *increased* the amount I drink, especially coffee made from beans with a high polyphenol content. I am careful with it though – I don't drink caffeinated coffee past 2pm as it disrupts my sleep and I only buy organic coffee from reputable brands that also check for mould and mycotoxins (see page 193). I'd rather pay a bit more for a delicious, premium brew with no added nasties.

Coffee is a plant food. It comes from fermented beans and, as far as I'm concerned, it happily sits in the 'superfood' category when it comes to health. I'm not alone in this viewpoint: in 2016, the WHO reversed its opinion of coffee from being a possible carcinogen to saying it either has no effect or can even 'reduce the risk of five different types of cancer', including uterine and liver cancers (significant, as coffee is processed via the liver). A year later, the *BMJ* published a meta-analysis of over 200 studies, concluding that coffee is positively good for us – as long as we aren't pregnant (UK government guidelines recommend a maximum of 200mg of caffeine a day while pregnant – around one strong cup of coffee). Those who drink three or more cups a day were found to have a reduced risk of some of our deadliest diseases, including chronic liver disease, Parkinson's and leukaemia, to name a few. Interestingly, each additional cup of coffee drunk a day was shown to reduce our risk of type 2 diabetes by a further 7 per cent (personally, I'd draw the line at three cups of the strong stuff a day).

In one massive American study of over half a million men and women, drinking 4 to 5 cups of coffee a day was strongly associated with living longer – 12 per cent longer for men and 7 per cent longer for women. This was true even for decaffeinated coffee, indicating that it's not the caffeine that's having a protective effect here. Coffee doesn't just contain caffeine – there are many other bio-actives in each cup which might help explain this, including the bitter-tasting polyphenol called chlorogenic acid. This powerful phytochemical is linked to improved cardiovascular health and weight loss. Other polyphenols also help lower blood pressure and boost our nitric oxide levels (which is a good thing). In coffee, the polyphenols help reduce some of the jittery side effects of caffeine, making high polyphenolic coffee a good option for those who get jumpy after a few flat whites. I often mix caff with decaf and make a half-and-half brew, as I enjoy the mule-like kick coffee gives me, but more often need a slightly calmer energy fix. I also prefer more lightly roasted coffee beans for a smoother, sweeter flavour, which also gives me more chlorogenic acid as this gets reduced the longer the beans are roasted. I've listed a few of my favourite coffee suppliers on page 310. Green coffee beans contain the highest levels of chlorogenic acid, followed by a light roast, medium roast and lastly darkly roasted coffee.

Perhaps due to its chlorogenic content, coffee drinking is also associated with longer telomere length, parts of our DNA that get shorter as we age (see page 48). The fact that drinking coffee has been shown to have a positive effect on telomere preservation is something of a breakthrough. Even drinking decaf has been shown to have a good effect. The American-backed National Health and Nutritional Examination Survey (NHANES) of over 5,000 adults found that, for each cup of coffee drunk, telomeres were increased by an average of 33.8 base pairs. We lose, on average, anywhere between 35 and 150 base pairs a year with age, so it could be that coffee drinkers can expect to enjoy a younger biological age when measured by length of their telomeres. Interestingly, a follow-up to this study looked at over 4,000 female nurses and found that those drinking three or more cups of coffee a day had the longest telomeres overall.

Mould and mycotoxins explained

One other important point to mention before leaving on a caffeine high is that of mould and mycotoxins. This is increasingly being raised as a point of potential concern for coffee lovers but, as is so often the case, the scare is not always supported by science. Mycotoxins are a type of mould or fungi that can be very harmful to health. They have been found in coffee beans, especially in the

What about instant coffee?

Interestingly, instant coffee holds its own in terms of polyphenol compounds – its benefits are pretty much equal to freshly ground coffee. But instant coffee contains twice as much acrylamide, a not-so-nice chemical formed during a reaction between amino acids and carbohydrates when heated, linked to cancer. On the plus side, instant coffee has around a third less caffeine and a far milder taste, making it a better choice for those who prefer a weaker brew or those who are caffeine-sensitive.

natural, green bean form before they're roasted. There are different kinds of mycotoxins, but the most studied are oachratoxin A (OTA) and aflatoxins (also associated with nuts, notably peanuts). A study in 2015 by researchers at the University of Valencia in Spain found that over half the samples tested contained aflatoxins, with OTA mainly found in instant coffee, but also in coffee capsules and decaffeinated coffee. The researchers concluded that, although mycotoxins were found to be present (in a few cases over permitted levels), their results were 'not alarming', although their work did raise questions on how levels could be better monitored and reduced in the future.

So why is there mould in our coffee and should we be more alarmed than the researchers seem to be? Mould occurs where there is humidity and there are many opportunities along the supply chain for coffee beans to become damp and encourage mycotoxins. The longer the beans are left green and unroasted, the more likely they are to become contaminated. While it's not considered a significant health risk (yet) for the majority of us, those with a chronic health condition such as kidney or liver disease (where coffee is broken down and processed in the body) should consider limiting their intake. Bear in mind though that, as we've seen, coffee brings a mass of health-protective benefits that may well mitigate any potential downside. It makes sense to buy from brands that are alive to the issue and can prove their beans have been thoroughly tested along every step of their journey, from cultivation to cup, stored correctly and freshly ground just before purchase. Once bought, all forms of coffee should be kept cool and dry, never in the fridge or freezer where higher humidity levels can encourage mould growth.

Consider spending a bit more on your coffee beans but drinking fewer cups, so the extra cost balances out.

My coffee buyers' guide

As a self-confessed coffee addict, here are my criteria when it comes to buying and brewing the best cup of coffee:

- Look for a few fundamentals on the label: organically certified, pesticide-free, mycotoxin-tested with a high polyphenol content. When buying decaf, look for the words 'water-process extraction' to ensure that the decaffeination process avoids traces of solvent residues inevitably left behind by chemical extraction.
- Buy whole beans and keep them in an airtight tin.
- Check the best before dates, and buy little and often to keep the beans fresh.

The health benefits of tea

We're a nation of tea drinkers here in the UK, sipping around 100 million cups each and every day (according to the UK Tea and Infusions Association), but is it good for us? The answer is a resounding yes – and it can be made even better for us when it comes to increasing healthspan depending on the type of tea and how we drink it. All tea (from green tea to builders' brew) comes from the leaves of the *Camellia sinensis* bush. All types contain useful levels of plant polyphenols (antioxidants), alongside other nutrients, and studies consistently show the more tea we drink, the lower our risk of death from all causes, including heart disease and stroke. Black tea has also been shown to reduce the LDL form of cholesterol (see page 127) and helps lower blood pressure. The latest research shows polyphenols in tea supporting the growth of good gut bugs in the digestive tract, which may then help repair the lining of the digestive system.

The difference between teas comes down to the way the leaves are harvested and dried. Green tea leaves are heated soon after picking, which prevents the leaf from oxidising and turning brown. Matcha is a type of green tea (again, from the same plant), where the leaves get pulverised to make the traditional bright green powder. The amount of caffeine in tea depends on how it's been processed: green tea contains around 11–25mg of caffeine per gram, which is similar to coffee. Matcha tea has around 19–44mg of caffeine per gram. But tea does not give us quite the same coffee buzz as it also contains L-theanine, an amino acid which helps soothe the nervous system by supporting the brain-calming chemicals gamma-aminobutyric acid (GABA), dopamine and serotonin. L-theanine also crosses the blood–brain barrier to increase alpha activity in the brain, helping us feel more relaxed and focused. So if you like the pick-me-up from coffee but find it makes you a bit too wired, switching to green or matcha tea could be the answer.

Both green tea and matcha tea are high in antioxidants, notably the catechin epigallocatechin-3-gallate, with the highest levels found in matcha tea. Because matcha uses the whole leaf ground up, it also contains a more complete array of plant polyphenols. When we drink matcha, we're actually swallowing the whole leaf dissolved in hot water, whereas with black or green teas, we steep the leaves before discarding them. So if you're drinking tea for a health fix, matcha is your best bet – as long as you don't mind its very 'green' grassy taste.

Black or white?

Several studies seem to suggest that adding milk to tea reduces the bioavailability of tea polyphenols, reducing its antioxidant effects, but this depends on the amount and type of milk added. Overall, whole milk has less of an effect and a splash of milk appears to have no effect whatsoever. This may be due to low-fat milk having fewer fat-soluble antioxidants, lowering overall levels in your cuppa. Interestingly, adding sugar to milky tea actually prevents catechin–milk protein interaction – but that's not a good enough reason to add sugar! Also, bear in mind that most of us drink tea as refreshment, not thinking about topping up our antioxidant levels, so I consider milk in tea to be a non-issue – add some if you like it.

Herb teas

Over the years I've got more into drinking herb teas and making my own blends. Herbs have so many therapeutic properties, as well as tasting great! They can also be powerfully pro-ageing and help with easing common ailments. I grow many tea-friendly herbs in my garden or on my kitchen windowsill and have a large pot of fresh mint growing right outside the kitchen door, ready to snip a few leaves for an after-dinner cup of digestive settlement. Cheap, easy, tasty and effective, mint is prolific in the summer months, so I cut and dry as much as I can then, storing the dried leaves in a tin to take me through the winter. I do the same with other common culinary herbs: thyme, sage, lemon balm ... and the botanicals that I don't grow (such as hibiscus and liquorice sticks) I buy in bulk online (see page 311 for my favourite suppliers). I make single or mixed-herb blends in a teapot and, instead of buying herb tea bags, I stock up with paper drawstring tea bags from a herbal supplier and make my own blends – so much cheaper, potentially more potent ... and more fun! These make thoughtful gifts too as you can tailor their contents according to need. Just keep in mind that all herbs contain therapeutic compounds, which although helpful in small amounts, can also interact with some prescription medications (such as thyroid drugs, sedatives, selective serotonin reuptake inhibitors (SSRIs) and blood thinners), so check with your doctor if you have any concerns.

These are some of my favourite herbs for tea:

Chamomile: proven to help us sleep, research shows that chamomile can also help regulate blood sugars and ease symptoms of PMS. I drink chamomile tea when I need to feel calmer. It's also good after dinner as a stomach soother and a way to unwind from the stresses of the day. Freshly dried chamomile flowers are readily available to buy in bulk (or grow your own).

Fennel seeds: so simple and effective, fennel has been used for digestive issues for centuries, even being given to babies to ease colic. Simply steep a few fennel seeds in some hot water for a deliciously tasty stomach settler. Especially good after a heavy meal or if you feel bloated, fennel-seed tea has been shown to help ease IBS and other conditions affecting the gastrointestinal system. More recent studies show fennel seeds to be protective against oxidative damage that happens to our DNA as we age.

Ginger: a classic kitchen staple, I am never without a piece of fresh ginger root somewhere in my fridge. It also freezes well, so I buy in bulk, peel and then freeze in chunks, ready to use (it's easy to grate then too). It is powerfully antioxidant and very good for settling all kinds of nausea, from morning sickness to travel sickness and chemo-induced sickness (and even hangovers). Studies show that it can also improve blood-sugar control. I drink it with sage, lemon peel and a small amount of raw (local) honey at the first sign of a cold or sore throat – this combination never fails me.

Hibiscus: I discovered hibiscus tea in Kenya and often bring a bag back home with me whenever I'm over there staying with my eldest son, who lives in Nairobi. Made from the dried hibiscus flower, this tea has a fabulously deep pink colour and unique, floral flavour. Shown to significantly reduce blood pressure and cholesterol, it could be worth trying as a natural support for these conditions (though always discuss this with your doctor first). It's also absolutely delicious, hot or chilled over ice, either served on its own or with a squeeze of fresh lime or lemon and a hint of raw honey.

Lemon balm or lemon verbena: a powerful, yet calming pick-me-up, these lemony leaves are not only rich in antioxidants, but clinical studies have also shown this scented herbal leaf can help improve symptoms of depression and clinical anxiety, alongside insomnia, headaches and memory loss. I love the refreshing lemony flavour, and verbena tea (verveine) is very popular in France as an after-dinner digestif.

Liquorice: a personal favourite, liquorice also combines well with dried lemon peel, lemon balm and ginger. I buy bags of dried liquorice sticks and simply steep a piece in a mug of hot water to release its aniseed-like flavour. Used in many traditional medicines for helping with upset stomachs and upper-respiratory problems, herbalists may use liquorice for indigestion, acid reflux, peptic ulcers, *H. pylori* (see page 210), asthma, strep throat, diabetes, bacterial and viral infections. It's a highly active botanical, even slowing the growth of cancer cells in test tubes and animals. Its main active component is glycyrrhizin, an anti-inflammatory and potent antioxidant, with studies showing it can help improve eczema and menopausal hot flushes. Large amounts can increase the stress hormone cortisol and are not recommended during pregnancy or for those with high blood pressure or taking blood thinners.

Peppermint: a wonderful digestive, peppermint is also highly antioxidant, with potent antibacterial and antiviral properties. Peppermint is also useful for relieving indigestion, nausea and IBS – it's one of my regular go-to teas. Acting as a mild muscle relaxant, drinking this tea before bed can help you get a good night's sleep as well as being a potentially helpful pain reliever for tension headaches. Peppermint oil is also effective against the bacteria in the mouth that cause bad breath (one reason why it's so popular in chewing gum and mints). As the plant's leaves contain its oil glands, peppermint leaf tea can help with this also. I drink it after dinner if I've been drinking alcohol, as it helps increase my fluid intake and lessens the effects of the alcohol. During the day, inhaling the oil (even breathing in the vapour from a steaming mug of peppermint tea) has been shown to increase alertness and cognitive function.

Rooibos: this is increasing in popularity among those looking for a more traditional 'tea'-tasting cuppa that's a caffeine-free herbal option, unrelated to black or green tea. Also known as 'red bush' tea, traditional rooibos is made by fermenting the leaves, which turns them a reddish brown (so it's not ideal for those with histamine sensitivity), but you can find green rooibos, which is not fermented (it also contains more antioxidants). Research shows that all forms of rooibos can lower blood pressure and cholesterol levels, as well as inhibit the formation of osteoclasts. These are cells that lead to the breaking down of bone and issues such as osteoporosis. I first discovered rooibos tea in South Africa, where it is hugely popular, but its reach is spreading far and wide and you'll now find all kinds of brands in many supermarkets. It's usually drunk black, but I do like to add a splash of milk sometimes. It's also good for making iced tea and frappes.

Sage: from the same plant family as mint, this herb also makes a wonderfully simple yet powerful tisane. A single sage leaf steeped in hot water creates a potent brew packed with bug-busting antioxidants. It is especially rich in rosmarinic acid, shown in test tube and animal studies to reduce inflammation and stabilise blood sugar.

Studies also show sage to be helpful for improving age-related cognitive decline. It is excellent for fighting coughs, colds and flu bugs, and I gargle with warm sage tea at the first tingle of a sore throat. Sage tea also makes an excellent natural mouthwash.

The 'Demon' Drink

I can't write a chapter about drinking without including a word or more about alcohol, particularly in relation to midlife wellness and ageing. Overall, studies seem to come down in favour of drinking a small amount of alcohol, reducing our risk of heart disease, stroke, dementia and possibly even type 2 diabetes; but some studies have also linked alcohol with a reduced lifespan, with cancers related to alcohol as the top causes of death (these studies included heavy drinkers). The more we drink, the greater the risk of disease and we should never drink so much that we overload our livers with more than they can process at any one time. Putting it bluntly, alcohol is a poison. Its main psychoactive ingredient is ethanol – the substance that gets us drunk. Ethanol also blurs the communication between brain cells, which is why we should never make any important decision after a few drinks! The liver is the main organ of detoxification and is the workhorse when it comes to metabolising ethanol.

Our relationship with alcohol is often complex and, by the time we reach midlife, we'll have settled into some established patterns of drinking. We may have even found the amount that we drink on a regular basis has crept ever-upwards over the years. I know that was true for me, especially during the dreadful lockdown years when I found myself opening that bottle of wine earlier in the day

– and frequently finishing it, even if I was alone. Not a good habit and not one I was proud of. It was while I was reviewing a fasting clinic that I not only stopped my nightly wine habit, but took a clear, hard look at whether or not I actually wanted to drink alcohol at all. Fasting meant not only no solid food, but no caffeine, sugar – or alcohol. I found I actually missed tea more than alcohol, so decided to continue with my abstinence on my return to the real world. Fasting is not only a way to take a break from poor eating habits but the mental clarity that comes with it often sparks a new way of living. I ended up being entirely alcohol-free for eight months, which I found both easy and enjoyable as there are so many great zero-alcohol alternatives out there. Even major gin brands are now making 0% spirits and there are good alcohol-free wines popping up in supermarkets too. I also drank a lot more gut-friendly kombucha . . . My clearer head was a morning bonus but I was struck by just how much alcohol surrounds us wherever we look, from endless adverts showing us happy times fuelled by drink, to the accepted culture of regular drinking. Alcohol can be enjoyable for sure, but it's also a pervasive poison and we shouldn't underestimate its reach. Today, I enjoy the occasional glass of wine or tequila and soda when out with friends, but I never drink alcohol when I'm alone and rarely have more than one or two glasses.

If you are drinking alcohol, it's better to do so regularly as the body cleverly adapts to patterns of behaviour as a way of coping. I've spoken to doctors who reveal they wouldn't say so publicly, but drinking alcohol every day is better for us than being 'dry' all week and saving up our 'units' for overindulgence at the weekend. However, this is definitely not an excuse to crack open the alcohol daily, unless you're disciplined enough to limit yourself solely to a single small glass of wine (125ml, about 12% alcohol), with food, each evening. The way we process alcohol is also influenced by our genes – some of us are able to process it better than others. And don't forget, alcohol is addictive and triggers carb cravings, so you're more likely to tuck into the toast or sugary snacks after drinking. If it's adversely affecting your life, or you can't live without it, you may well have a problem with alcohol dependence or alcoholism. If this strikes a chord, I've included a few resources to reach out to for help on page 306.

Some types of alcohol are definitely better for us than others. Red wine tops the leader board as it's high in healthy antioxidants, including resveratrol. Found mainly in grape skins, resveratrol is a plant compound known as a phytoalexin, a natural antibiotic designed to protect the plant from attacks from fungi, UV radiation, predatory bugs and bacteria. It would seem that resveratrol can give our human cells similar protective benefits too. Resveratrol also shows promise as an anti-cancer supplement, switching on the cancer-protective intracellular signalling while also suppressing the expression of NAF-1, transferring proteins that can stimulate cancer growth. Resveratrol has also been shown to stimulate apoptosis and autophagy (I hope you made a note of these two important cellular health activities we discussed on pages 55 and 57). I no longer drink red wine daily, limiting myself to the odd glass or two, but having studied the data, I do now take resveratrol as a supplement. Red wine also contains anthocyanins, antioxidants found in colourful fruit and veg (notably purple fruits, such as blueberries). This is why red wine is better for us than white, as although both are made from black grapes, the skins are left on during the winemaking process, which is what gives red wine its colour and flavour.

Although red wine confers certain health benefits, when it comes to sugar in wine, champagne wins the day. The least-sugar options are Brut Nature with up to 3g sugar per litre and Extra Brut with up to 6g per litre (the word 'brut' indicates the driest types of champagne). The main sugars in wine are glucose and fructose, and a single glass of port can contain up to 100g of sugar. Dessert or pudding wines are also massively high in sugars – you might as well eat fermented sugar cubes. Unfortunately, cheaper, mass-produced wines also have higher sugar levels as they are made on an industrial scale and some wineries use tricks such as adding more sugar to disguise the taste of poor-quality, sour grapes. No wine can be truly sugar-free, but there are increasing numbers of lower-sugar options popping up on the shelves.

The downside to lower-sugar wines is that they tend to be higher in alcohol. So our choice as consumers comes down to alcohol versus sugar levels. Alcohol is listed on labels as a percentage of ABV, or alcohol by volume. When I'm choosing wine, I try to stick to 12 per cent or less, not always easy when it comes to my favourite red Burgundy. But winemakers are becoming more aware of the low-sugar trend and choice is increasing. Anything below 12 per cent ABV is considered a low-alcohol wine. Typically, a dry red wine, such as Cabernet Sauvignon, is low-sugar with less than 2g per glass, but is likely to be between 13 and 15 per cent alcohol. I also look for the words 'organic' or 'biodynamic' on the label, as these tend to be better-quality wines from smaller producers who make their wine with a bit more care and less reliance on chemical horticulture (and the good news is you can increasingly find these in some of the lower-cost supermarkets, such as Lidl, now too). Grapes are not washed before they are crushed, so any toxic pesticide or other residues on the grape skins will end up in the bottle.

Also, keep in mind that all wine and champagnes are fermented, so are high in histamine and will not suit those who need to avoid foods or any drink (including beers) made by fermentation.

Cocktail time

Although all spirits are very high in alcohol, being distilled they're also virtually sugar-free. This doesn't make them a low-calorie option though, as alcohol contains even more calories per gram than sugar. With the exception of whisky perhaps, we also rarely drink spirits on their own and their mixers are often very high in sugar (or artificial sweeteners, which, as we saw on page 179, are often not a healthy option). Vodka is classically cited as being the 'purest' form of spirit and least likely to give us a hangover, but its wellness fame is being supplanted by the claims now being made about tequila.

The noise around tequila comes from the compounds in agave, a Mexican cactus, not the alcohol itself, but the benefits of this are most likely to have been broken down by the time the spirit reaches the bottle. Tequila is made from fermented agave juice, with high-end blue, silver or white tequilas typically coming from Mexico where they're made with 100 per cent fermented agave. Raw agave contains anti-inflammatory compounds and gut-friendly prebiotics, but whether these end up in our margaritas is debatable. The good news is that tequila is sugar-free, with one 42g shot of pure tequila giving us around 100Kcals and zero carbs.

Deciding what we drink is every bit as important as what we eat. Many drinks are positively beneficial (essential), so make sure you have a supply of the better options on hand. Invest in a water filter (jugs are basic, but fine) and do look at adding a daily dose of electrolytes. These make all the difference to how you feel. Look out for the wonderful array of alcohol-free options around now – my drinks cupboard is filled with all kinds of delicious alternatives within easy reach whenever I fancy a zero-alcohol G&T or cocktail. I served botanical cocktails at my 60th birthday party – mine made with 0% gin; it tasted every bit as good and I was up with the lark feeling great (many of my guests, not so much).

Healthy hacks
- Work out how much water you need to be drinking daily and keep a water jug/bottle on your kitchen counter or desk as a visual reminder.
- Read labels for hidden sugars, especially when it comes to so-called health or 'energy' drinks. Fruit juice is very high in sugar, so always drink juices well diluted with water, if at all.
- Review the amount of alcohol you're drinking. Make it an occasional pastime, not a daily pleasure, unless you're disciplined enough to make it a single, small glass of wine daily (and very rarely any more than this).

CHAPTER 7

Healthy Ageing Lies in Your Gut Health

I guess we all know by now that looking after our good gut bugs has to be a priority in life, both for our physical and mental well-being. And there are so many easy health hacks we can do daily to support this. The small amount of effort we make here can dramatically change how we feel, not only with improved digestion, fewer digestive issues and better outcomes for IBS, reflux, leaky gut (see page 211) and all the rest, but also for the immune system (up to 80 per cent of which originates in the gut) and improved mental health, due to the gut–brain axis. There's a very powerful connection between our hormones and brain neurotransmitters (chemical messengers that support the brain, such as dopamine, serotonin, GABA and so on), all of which are controlled by what happens in the gut. The gut is connected to the brain via the vagus nerve, the largest nerve in the body that touches almost every important part of the body from the backside to the brain. Neurotransmitters travel at lightning speed up and down this internal superhighway, influencing our every thought, mood and emotion. This is why recognising the impact of gut health on how we *feel* is so fantastically important. We're also learning more about the gut–hormone, gut–skin and gut–sleep axes too; in fact, there's no part of the body the micro-biome doesn't influence.

The gut microbiome has been described as a newly found vital organ of the body (the others being the brain, heart, lungs, liver and kidneys). The term 'microbiome' refers to the trillions of bacteria, fungi and other microbes, all of which play a vital part in the way we digest what we eat and drink, plus so much more besides. We can support it by eating foods that make the good gut bugs thrive and reducing the foods that encourage an overgrowth of the bad bugs. I like to think of the microbiome as a bit of a battlefield – we need to equip our good gut bugs with the nourishment they need to multiply and overcome the 'enemy' bad guys. We do this with plant fibres (good gut bugs love to feed on these) and fermented foods such as yoghurt, kefir and kimchi (more on those in a moment); whereas the bad bugs feed on sugars, so every time we eat something high in sugar, we're equipping the enemy . . . According to Dr William Davis, the American cardiologist who calls modern wheat 'a perfect, chronic poison' and is the author of many bestsellers, including the brilliant book *Super Gut*, lots of sugar in our diets is virtually a guaranteed set-up for significantly poorer gut health.

An imbalance of good and bad gut bugs is called gut dysbiosis, something we want to avoid for many good reasons. When dysbiotic microbes travel from the colon up into the small intestine they create something called small intestinal bacterial overgrowth (SIBO). This is something that can be detected with a DIY breath test at home if you're concerned it could be causing your gut-health problems (there are a number available online, or ask your GP to refer you to an NHS gastroenterologist). SIBO is surprisingly common, and can show up as IBS, sleep disturbances, skin rashes, allergies, depression, unexplained pain, restless legs syndrome and menstrual disturbances – you name it, SIBO can be a cause, such is the pervasive reach and influence of these microscopic bad actors. SIBO has also been shown to increase the incidence of *H. pylori*, a pernicious bug that can be helpful in small amounts (especially with reflux issues), but when it proliferates out of control can lead to rosacea, stomach ulcers and even some kinds of cancer. More recently, it has been linked with stomach and pancreatic cancers, type 2 diabetes and Parkinson's disease. *H. pylori* lowers stomach acid, which is not a good thing, and if you are diagnosed with it, some of the more natural remedies shown to help include *Nigella sativa* (black cumin seeds), mastic gum (the resin from a Mediterranean tree), vitamin C and N-acetyl cysteine (NAC – a powerful disruptor of bacterial biofilm, another hard-to-treat collective of bad-boy superbugs).

Our microbiomes control just so much of who we are and how our bodies function. Let's explore a few links with gut health, starting with how much we weigh.

Gut health and weight gain

Gut dysbiosis leads to us putting on more weight than we should. We know this from studies looking at identical twins, genetically the same in every way except for what's happening within their microbiomes. When gut microbes from a bigger twin were transferred to their smaller twin, they too gained weight, without changing what they ate. Such is the power of these mighty microbes.

Gut health and digestive issues

The microbiome controls intestinal disorders such as IBS, IBD, bloating, stomach cramps, acid reflux, indigestion, wind and more. This is because the bad gut bugs produce gas and other compounds that not only make us feel uncomfortable, but create small holes in our gut walls, leading to leaky gut and potentially triggering intolerances to foods such as gluten and lactose. Instead of switching to a 'free-from' restricted diet to screen out these foods, a healthier strategy is to help the gut repair these perforations, so food intolerances disappear, or at least become much less of an issue. Some of the best probiotic bacteria (one kind of good gut bug) are *Bifidobacteria* and *Lactobacilli*, found in yoghurt and kefir, which help seal the gaps between intestinal cells, strengthening the wall of the microbiome. These species of bacteria also stop the bad bugs that lead to disease in general from sticking to the sides of the intestines. Something as simple as eating a little plain, live yoghurt every day can have a big impact, and has even been shown to decrease lactose intolerance.

Gut health and heart disease

Beneficial gut bugs help protect our hearts by supporting the 'good' form of cholesterol and blood fats. By contrast, the bad bugs produce something called trimethylamine N-oxide (TMAO), a chemical that leads to blocked arteries and may cause heart attacks or stroke. *Lactobacilli* has been shown to help regulate cholesterol and reduce levels of TMAO, in turn reducing our overall risk of heart disease.

Gut health and menopause

A specific collection of bacteria (and their genes) in the gut have been found to influence oestrogen, and this is termed the 'oestrobolome'. New studies show that certain gut microbes play an important role in how our bodies utilise oestrogen, by influencing oestrogen-metabolising enzymes called beta-glucuronidases. These small but mighty substances convert oestrogens into their active forms, so they are better able to enter the blood circulation and reach tissues all around the body. It's fascinating to realise that by promoting certain species of gut bugs, we can help make a significant impact on our meno-pausal (and perimenopausal) symptoms.

When we lose oestrogen (either through chronological body ageing or medical treatment), the delicate balancing act going on within the oestrobolome is affected. This results in changes to how the body uses what little oestrogen it has left and is being linked to the increased risk of weight gain, cancers (including breast cancer) and degenerative conditions such as type 2 diabetes and coronary heart disease.

The best foods to eat to support a healthy oestrobolome include even small amounts of fibre from vegetables, whole grains, nuts and seeds as well as some of the fruits that are lower in sugars (apples, berries of all kinds and stone fruits such as plums and apricots). Other foods being investigated for their oestrobolome-supporting activity include those rich in phytoestrogens, such as soya beans, tofu and tempeh. Probiotic supplements may also have the potential to help out here, with *Lactobacilli* supplemen-tation being investigated for a potential link with breast cancer prevention. It may be that in the future, specific probiotic supple-ments will be recommended for helping to reduce the risk of all kinds of oestrogen-related health issues, especially around the time of the menopause.

Gut health and the brain

Several types of bacteria in the gut produce neurotransmitters. Notable among these is serotonin, a naturally antidepressant neurotransmitter that we predominantly make in the gut. Studies show that those with a disrupted microbiome, due to the stress hormone cortisol, taking antibiotics or overloading with sugars, are more likely to suffer mental health-issues, ranging from mild anxiety, stress and depression to more severe conditions such as bipolar disorder. One strain of *Bifidobacterium longum* called NCC3001 has been shown to be especially protective here. Another superstar is *Lactobacillus reuteri*, one of my favourite good gut bugs (found in yoghurt as well as specifically in some probiotics – look out for it on the label). *L. reuteri* has been shown to uniquely trigger the production of oxytocin in the brain, otherwise known as the 'love bug', as it surges when we feel love towards something – another person, a beautiful view, even our dogs. It's the hormone that's released at orgasm, giving us a surge of feel-good emotions. Sex supports better gut health! Smaller amounts of oxytocin produce feelings of connectedness and empathy. It's a natural wonder. Animal studies also show that supplements of *L. reuteri* increase collagen, promote wound-healing, help with weight control, as well as reducing the stress hormone cortisol. You'll find it in meat and dairy products, especially cheeses such as Cheddar, Gruyère and Parmesan.

Your Essential Gut Allies

When it comes to getting more of the good gut bugs in our micro-biomes to crowd out the bad, there are three important allies:

Prebiotics

These are dietary fibres that feed our good gut bugs, much like a fertiliser feeding plants. One example is inulin, a fibre found in plants such as chicory, dandelion greens, onions, leeks and arti-chokes, which we don't digest well in the stomach so it travels on to feed our microbes, allowing them to thrive. Galactooligosaccharides (GOS) and fructooligosaccharides (FOS) are also prebiotics found in some specific gut health supplements. Once fed, our good gut bugs make nutrients to support our microbiomes, such as the short-chain fatty acid butyrate. Prebiotic supplements are a way to fast-track to better gut health and can be taken daily. Look out for brands such as Bimuno (made with GOS) and any form of butyrate, which specifically helps build a stronger gut barrier to keep out bad bacteria and other noxious microbes. Butyrate is an essential ally for anyone with leaky gut or food intolerances (it's also found in butter, hence its name; another reason why I spread plenty of butter on my bread).

Probiotics

Probiotics are the live bacteria found in fermented food and drinks, such as yoghurt, kefir, kombucha, sauerkraut and properly fermented pickles (not just those made with a quick splash of vine-gar). When buying any of these, make sure they're not pasteurised as this form of heat treatment kills the good bugs. Check that your yoghurt says it is 'bio' or 'live' if you're buying it (homemade fermented foods and drinks are also a great option – see below). A few foods are both pre- and probiotic, such as cheese, kefir and sauerkraut, as these contain both beneficial bacteria *and* the food they need to proliferate – a double whammy of goodness. You can also buy probiotic supplements to top up your daily supply, but because beneficial bacteria only live for a few days in the gut, you do need to take them regularly for best effect.

Postbiotics

Postbiotics are becoming more talked about as we discover that our microbes produce additional, helpful bacteria to further support our gut health. They include short-chain fatty acids (such as butyrate), enzymes and bacterial lysates. Part of their function is to make anti-inflammatory messengers called cytokines that lower inflammation in the body and support our immune systems. Those with IBD tend to have lower levels of short-chain fatty acids, and studies have found that for those with Crohn's disease and some allergies, such as eczema, taking 4g of butyrate daily for eight weeks saw improvement (and even remission) in over half of the participants.

Add in the 5 Ks for Gut Health

No, I don't mean dust off your running shoes, this is all about adding in these dietary 5 Ks . . . One of the biggest changes I've made to my diet over the years has been adding in many more fermented foods. If you're new to this, take it slowly. A sudden influx of even beneficial bacteria can cause digestive upsets!

**Start with very small amounts and
gradually increase as your gut microbes
get used to their new-found friends.**

Kamut

Otherwise known as sourdough, kamut doesn't actually contain probiotics, as bread is cooked which kills the microbes, but it uses beneficial *Lactobacillus* bacteria in the process of making it. It does have digestive benefits though, as the fermentation process breaks down gluten (many who are gluten intolerant discover they can eat sourdough bread made with wheat). It is easier to digest too, as my own father can attest when he queried why the toast I served him at breakfast did not have him reaching for his regular indigestion remedy. This unique fermentation process also increases the bioavailability of the bread's vitamins and minerals, making it naturally more nutritious.

Real sourdough bread takes time to make – it can't be rushed as the flour and water need several days for the wild yeasts to properly leaven the dough. Unfortunately, its ever-increasing popularity has seen the rise of 'sourfaux' – bread labelled as sourdough but commercially made using shortcuts such as ascorbic acid, vinegar and oil which hasten its production time (so it costs less to make). A 2018 study by *Which?* magazine revealed that out of 19 sourdough loaves being sold in supermarkets, only 4 were traditionally made. If you're buying sourdough, look for a few clues on the label. The real deal will contain just three ingredients – flour, water and salt (these may be labelled as 'starter culture') – and nothing else, except perhaps different types of grain or a sprinkling of seeds for some speciality types. If a bread contains yeast or sugar, it is not genuine sourdough.

Real sourdough is also full of holes, caused by the natural fermentation process.

Sourdough tends to go off quickly, so check its best before date (anything longer than a few days or so is suspicious). It's best stored wrapped in a clean tea towel, cloth bread bag or wooden bread box. Don't keep it in the fridge, as the cold air will make the bread go hard. I buy my sourdough from a local baker, slice it up and freeze it as soon as I get home, ready to toast as needed straight from the freezer.

Kefir

Possibly my favourite ferment of all, the word kefir comes from the Turkish word *keyif*, meaning 'feeling good' and I love it for its yoghurty tang and superb versatility. Similar to yoghurt, but much runnier and slightly fizzy (due to the carbon dioxide released during fermentation), kefir can be drunk neat or thickened to make kefir yoghurt. Made from kefir grains (or powdered grains), it's packed with *Lactobacillus* probiotics, including *L. parakefiri* and *L. brevis* alongside unusual yeasts, and it has unusual antimicrobial activity that can neutralise pathogenic (bad) bacteria. This is why it is often recommended to help gastrointestinal upsets and can be helpful to treat candida and other unwanted microbial overgrowths.

Fermented dairy products, such as yoghurt and kefir, have also been shown to have anti-tumour properties and appear to act as antioxidants, supporting a stronger immune system. Real kefir is always made with animal milk, as its microbes use lactose (milk sugars) to grow. In fact, there is so little lactose left in the end product, most people who are lactose intolerant find they can have kefir without any problems. Purists argue there is no such thing as coconut or water 'kefirs', which may well have beneficial probiotic bacteria, but not the same potency or probiotic strains as genuine kefir made with animal milk (such as cow, goat or sheep's milk). You'll always find kefir in my fridge and I tend to drink it with brunch, although any time of day is good, to be honest. I make sure to buy some of the local stuff whenever I travel, treating my gut bugs to new diversities (it also helps to protect against 'traveller's tum' and avoid stomach bugs too).

Kimchi

This is a traditional Korean fermented relish, often quite spicy, made with chopped-up veggies with garlic, chilli, ginger and other spices. The starting point is some kind of cabbage, such as napa or Chinese cabbage, and the best kinds are left for many days (often weeks or months) to ferment in their own juices, allowing the beneficial microbes to multiply. A single dessertspoonful of kimchi can contain around a billion good gut bugs, often from the lactic acid family, likely to include *L. reuteri* and *rhamnosus* bacteria, especially good for female pelvic health and happy neurotransmitters. Kimchi adds a delicious acidy tang to savoury dishes and, once you get the taste for it, you'll find yourself adding it to just about everything from salads and sandwiches, to grilled meats and cheese dishes. It is a very healthy addition and cheap and easy to make at home too (see my website for a video on how to make it: lizearlewellbeing.com/healthy-food/healthy-recipes/lizs-larder/how-to-make-kimchi).

Kombucha

I've been making kombucha at home for decades, long before it became a trend. Back in the day, it was seen as a strange, slightly fizzy tea that weird people (like me) made in their airing cupboards. Perhaps because it looks so odd, to the uninitiated it can seem pretty peculiar, but appearances belie its powerful gut-friendly benefits. To make kombucha you first need a symbiotic culture of bacteria and yeast, known as a SCOBY. It looks like a rubbery pancake and can vary from the size of a small saucer to the largest one I've seen, around 2m in diameter, used for making the Liz Earle Wellbeing kombucha by British brand Mighty Brew. This particular gigantic beauty is now well over 20 years old and still going strong. That's because kombucha is a 'living' ferment, growing a SCOBY 'baby' every ten days or so that needs to be peeled away to start a new batch of brew.

A SCOBY needs a starter mixture of tea and sugar to grow and, when making kombucha, some are horrified by the amount of sugar that's dissolved into the black tea. But this is where the SCOBY works its magic – feeding off the sugar to ferment the liquid tea and turn it into a powerful probiotic drink. The end result is a drink that's actually very low in sugar. It's simple to make and delicious to drink, once you get used to the slightly vinegary taste. Kombucha can be flavoured with herbs and other botanicals (elderflower and lemon are two favourites I drink whenever I'm looking for a healthier juice or wine alternative) and drinking a small glass every day is a healthy habit that's great for replenishing a wide range of beneficial microbes, often including *Bacillus coagulans* or *Komagataeibacter* species, together with *Akkermansia*, the gut bug associated with weight loss. Each batch of kombucha is likely to be slightly different though (especially when homemade) as the SCOBY absorbs airborne bacteria and yeasts to turn them into good gut bugs. Pure alchemy. (See my website for a kombucha recipe if you're interested in making it at home: lizearlewellbeing.com/healthy-food/healthy-recipes/drinks/how-to-make-kombucha.)

Kraut

Otherwise known as sauerkraut, in its simplest form kraut is just plain cabbage, finely sliced and fermented in salt water. The easiest (and cheapest) kind of fermented food to make at home, using a finely sliced cabbage, a handful of rock or sea salt topped up with water in a large jar, it takes just two to three days for the good gut bugs to start to proliferate. You can add all kinds of flavourings – I like to make mine by adding garlic cloves, chopped ginger root and fennel seeds, but you can add whatever flavours you like. Lemon, caraway seeds and dill also work well. Sauerkraut tends to contain *Lactobacillus* strains of bacteria, including *L. brevis* and *L. plantarum*. If you buy sauerkraut, be sure it is the real deal: properly fermented and not pasteurised (which kills the bacteria).

Cacao

Although spelled with a C and not a K, cacao deserves a special mention here as it also positively impacts the gut microbiome. A study conducted by Louisiana State University researchers found that the fibre in cacao feeds healthy gut bacteria such as *Bifidobacteria* and *Lactobacilli*. You might not think that a cup of cocoa contains much fibre, but it has enough of the specific kind to support better gut health, strengthen the immune system and support insulin resistance. Cacao may even help correct disruptions to the microbiome caused by chronic stress – not to say that every time you are feeling anxious you should emotionally eat chocolate, but a comforting cup of cocoa sweetened with a little stevia or raw honey? Yes!

> **When *not* to eat**
>
> Supporting our gut microbiomes is more than just what we eat and drink. When *not* to ingest anything is also important. Studies show that intermittent fasting or TRE (see page 174) is a crucial part of better gut health. When I interviewed award-winning bestselling medical doctor and author Dr Jason Fung, for my podcast in 2023, I was astonished to hear that intermittent fasting provides as much as 70 per cent of the value when it comes to gut health, managing insulin resistance and losing weight. That's a staggering statistic – and a practice that's so simple to do. Definitely a healthy habit to get into.

Gut Health Supplements

In addition to fermented foods and drinks, there are a number of other specific gut-friendly supplements that I think are worth considering.

Apple cider vinegar

Studies show that drinking a spoonful (5–10ml) of apple cider vinegar in a little water before meals can reduce insulin sensitivity (good for type 2 diabetes and weight control) as well as help acid reflux, by introducing more acid into the digestive tract. However, it can aggravate stomach ulcers and also dissolve tooth enamel (I drink mine through a straw to avoid this). Clinical research is limited, but blood glucose monitor tests confirm its effectiveness for some, and many swear by its power to improve their overall digestive health. I don't drink it all the time, but if I know I'm heading for a high-carb meal, I'll drink a glassful beforehand and feel better for it.

Probiotics

There are many hundreds of probiotic supplements on the market, ranging from powders to liquids and capsules (see page 314 for some of my favourites). Adding in a daily probiotic supplement can be especially helpful if you're feeling in need of some powerful gut-friendly TLC, alongside adding in fermented foods and plant fibre. Supplements are good, but they are no substitute for a healthy diet. When choosing a probiotic, look for the numbers of different strains it contains, as diversity of bacteria is now thought to be more important than the amount of colony-forming units (CFUs). This is how probiotics are labelled:

Genus: the group of bacteria, e.g. *Lactobacillus*
Species: the individual type of bacterium, e.g. *rhamnosus*
Strain: a number or letter identifying the precise bug, e.g. NCFM

As an example, you might see the words *Lactobacillus rhamnosus* NCFM, indicating the exact kind of probiotic, useful when searching for one that has been identified as helping a particular condition (in this case, reducing the risk of SIBO and even colon cancer).

Olive leaf extract

From the leaves of the olive tree, this extract contains an unusual active ingredient called oleuropein, a substance with good anti-inflammatory and antioxidant properties. Not only can olive leaf extract help regulate blood fats, and therefore cholesterol, interesting studies show it may help prevent damage to the dopamine receptors in the brain linked to Parkinson's disease, as well as lower blood pressure and support the immune system by its action within the gut microbiome.

Slippery elm

Extracted from the inner bark of the *Ulmus rubra* tree, otherwise known as red elm or India elm, native to Canada, Native Americans have used this slimy secretion mixed in water to soothe the stomach (it was later used by American soldiers to heal wounds during the American Revolution). Slippery elm is a demulcent, meaning that it has properties that can sooth irritations. Studies show that slippery elm stimulates the nerves in the gastrointestinal tract, so they secrete more of the mucus that protects its lining against gastric ulcers and excess acidity. This has been shown to help those with IBS and Crohn's disease, and it is often recommended by naturopaths treating all kinds of gut health disorders, including indigestion, as well as UTIs and sore throats.

Soil-based probiotics

Known in the trade as SBOs or soil-based organisms, these are bacteria that have been isolated from the earth. Soil is teeming with beneficial bacteria that live in the ground, helping plants grow healthy and strong, and they bring benefits to our bodies too. SBOs improve our gut health by populating our microbiomes with a wider range of naturally beneficial bacteria than we would otherwise get from modern-day foods. They're a lost art, as in ancient times we would have ingested them from foraged foods or crops eaten without thorough washing, heat treatment or food processing. I'm a big fan of SBOs as an additional support for gut health and especially like brands such as Microbz, that grow their probiotic cultures from ancient wild pastures (see Useful Resources on page 314).

Whey

This watery by-product of cheese-making is a pre-digested protein, meaning that it's easier for the body to break down and more quickly absorbed than other forms of protein, which is why it's often found in protein powders and supplements. It's a high-quality, inexpensive form of protein, helping to build muscle mass as we age, but, interestingly, also helps symptoms of IBD, reduces inflammation in the gut and lowers blood pressure. There are many different forms of whey supplements on the market (including protein powders) and you'll also find it in dairy products, notably cottage cheese, yoghurt and ricotta.

I tend to take my gut health supplements on an empty stomach and often switch between different types and brands to increase my gut health diversity.

The more variety the better – more is more!

Look after your good gut bugs and they will look after you; it really is that simple. This is especially important as we get older, as the chances are we'll all have damaged (or even wrecked) our microbiomes with a lifetime of poor eating habits, excessive amounts of sugar and alcohol, stress, emotional upsets and/or medications such as antibiotics. Recognising this – and taking action – is one of the simplest ways of giving our bodies a better second half. Whatever stage of life you're at, it's never too late to make a difference. Just a few simple changes, such as eating more fermented foods, adding in a prebiotic and/or probiotic supplement and practising intermittent fasting will make a discernible difference to how well you age.

Healthy hacks
- Eat a small amount of the '5 Ks' each day: keep your kitchen stocked with kamut (sourdough), kefir, kimchi, kraut and kombucha. Your gut will thank you for it.
- If you're prescribed antibiotics, always take a probiotic supplement alongside to support the gut (and no, this will not affect the antibiotic action). Take this as soon as you start the course and continue for at least a week afterwards.
- Give your gut a break: TRE (see page 174) allows the digestive system to rest and repair, giving our good gut bugs a chance to down tools from their daily activity and focus on replenishing themselves.

CHAPTER 8

Protecting the Brain

As well as lifespan we need to think about our healthspan. There's one thing I'm sure we all want and that's to age well, free from pain, immobility, cognitive decline and incapacity.

One of the simplest things we can do to support our myriad neurological pathways is to fix any nutritional deficiency. On a purely biochemical level, there are several proven ways to do this to support better brain health as we age. One of the most important, which I'll cover first, is the healthy brain fats.

Why Fish Fats Are Key

They say that fish feeds the brain and this is true, although specifically we're talking about the oils found in fatty (oily) fish, notably DHA. When it comes to building a better brain, DHA is the real winner. Multiple clinical trials have linked low levels of DHA with cognitive decline as well as shown that supplements can reverse the downward curve and even help prevent dementia. Eating fish itself is helpful, with one study that followed fish-eaters over a seven-year period showing that they had significantly less risk of developing Alzheimer's disease just by eating fish twice a week, compared to those who rarely ate any. Those aged between 65 and 69 showed the most benefit, with less improvement beyond the age of 70, presumably because by then, there's too much cerebral blood-vessel damage to repair. MRI scans show that those with the most DHA in their diets have the least damage to white matter hyperintensities, important parts of the brain where nerve fibres carry signals deep within our brains. DHA has also been shown to improve memory recall, even reducing memory loss in those with mild cognitive impairment. Prevention is better than cure, but this demonstrates the potential power of DHA to make a difference to the way we think in older age.

So should we eat more fish? Yes! Especially the oily kind (see page 154). Fish oil supplements are a useful, cheaper, alternative (I take DHA daily), but it's important to buy only from reputable and established brands using sustainably caught fish with contaminant testing carried out on each batch. You'll find some of my preferred brands on page 312. Personally, I look for supplements coming from whole-body fish (rather than just fish livers, such as cod liver oil), as body oil is naturally lower in environmental toxins than liver oil, due to the liver storing whatever the creature has ingested, an increasing issue in today's polluted waters. I'm also a fan of krill, a supplement made from the tiny crustaceans eaten by whales and penguins, to name a few that feed on these. Krill are a very rich source of both EPA and DHA omega-3 fatty acids, as well as being high in the powerful antioxidant astaxanthin (this is deep red in colour, which is why krill oil capsules are a pretty shade of pink). The jury is out as to whether krill is better than fish oil, or vice versa. Some studies suggest that krill is better absorbed, while others beg to differ. Krill does have the advantage of containing astaxanthin and may be more anti-inflammatory, so unless you're getting this from another source (for example, mixed in with a collagen supplement), krill probably has the edge. I think both forms of omega-3 supplementation are good. The main thing is to take at least one of them each and every day.

Vegan omega-3s

You'll have noticed that both forms of omega-3 supplements mentioned above are animal-derived, so is there an effective vegan or vegetarian option? The short answer is yes; the long (more complete) answer is no. Many plant-based eaters are advised to take flaxseed (linseed) oil to obtain their quota of omega-3 essential fats. However, flaxseed oil contains ALA, a form of omega-3 fatty acid that converts into the neuro-protective powerhouse that is DHA, but only in tiny amounts. It also breaks down into toxic compounds when heated, so should only ever be used cold and never for cooking.

Brain Boosters

Other important nutrients to support better brain health include choline (eggs are a brilliant source), turmeric, vitamin K, selenium and B-complex vitamins – notably folate and vitamin B12. These two B vitamins are especially helpful as they combine to help break down the amino acid homocysteine in the brain, identified as a strong risk factor for vascular dementia, brain atrophy (basically the shrivelling of the brain over time) and Alzheimer's disease (vegans and veggies, do make sure you're getting enough of these, especially vitamin B12, principally found in foods of animal origin).

Gingko biloba is another interesting botanical, worthy of a mention when it comes to protecting the ageing brain. Extracted from the fan-shaped leaves of an ancient tree native to East Asia, ginkgo was one of the few trees to withstand the devastation of the atomic bomb that fell on Hiroshima in 1945.

Ginkgo biloba seems able to confer its power and strength to us mortals when it comes to brain preservation. Its properties stem from extraordinarily high levels of antioxidants as well as an ability to significantly increase nitric oxide, protecting blood vessels, cells and guarding against DNA damage. Ginkgo biloba has also been shown to reduce dementia and improve memory, with a comprehensive review concluding that those taking it showed 'stabilising or slowing decline in cognition of subjects with cognitive impairment and dementia', when taken for 22–24 weeks. Perhaps due to its ability to increase blood flow to the brain, some studies also suggest it may lessen anxiety and can help treat symptoms of depression. It's also been used to help those who have experienced a stroke, although it may be contraindicated for those taking blood thinners, SSRIs and non-steroidal anti-inflammatory drugs (NSAIDs, such as ibuprofen and naproxen).

Ginkgo biloba is certainly something to consider adding to our brain health repertoire.

The Health Benefits of Magical Mushrooms

No, I'm not talking here about psychedelic 'magic mushrooms' or psilocybin, to give it the proper scientific name. I'm referring to the phenomenal 'nootropic' fungi that have been around since the dawn of time (longer, in fact, than we have), proven to have a physical effect on our physique and psyche. Nootropic means that something has an effect on our brains, and all mushrooms possess this unusual property. They're increasingly cropping up in powders, drinks, functional foods and supplements, each with their own unique and powerful characteristics. All mushroom varieties (even the everyday kind we cook with) are a rich source of vitamin D (the only non-animal food source), especially when they've been exposed to sunlight, as they synthesise vitamin D3 through their skin in much the same way we do. This is why I pop my mushrooms onto a sunny windowsill before cooking them. Mushrooms should always be eaten cooked, by the way, never raw, as heat breaks down their tough cellular structure, releasing proteins, B vitamins and minerals, as well as beta-glucans, soluble fibres that help stop us absorbing excess fats, naturally regulate cholesterol and can help with weight loss. Beta-glucans have also been shown to stimulate the immune system and can even help kill cancer cells.

Each variety of mushroom possesses several unique and different superpowers. These are some of the key players worth knowing about, with their benefits when it comes to brain health and more besides:

Chaga (*inonotus obliquus*)

Hailed as the mightiest mushroom of all for its antioxidant activity, chaga is especially rich in superoxide dismutase (SOD), an enzyme renowned for reducing free radical cell damage due to ageing (especially where ageing skin in concerned, helping combat fine lines, wrinkles and pigmentation). Originally found on Russian birch trees, where it takes at least 15 years to mature, chaga delivers a potent energy hit and is a good addition to tea or coffee when you need a pick-me-up (I add mine to decaf coffee for a lift without the jitters). Researchers in Japan have found that chaga boosts memory, as well as improving overall cognition.

Cordyceps (*cordyceps militaris* and *cordyceps sinensis*)

Popular in TCM, cordyceps shot to fame in the 1993 Chinese National Games when the women's running team broke nine world records and were accused of drug-taking, only for it to be discovered they'd been taking cordyceps, not steroids or other kinds of stimulants. Reputedly aphrodisiac (its nickname is Himalayan Viagra), ancient records reveal cordyceps as a time-honoured boost to female libido, and studies show it can also improve a guy's testicular dysfunction, as well as increase testosterone levels in both men and women. When it comes to the brain, cordyceps has an antidepressant effect, activating dopamine receptors, making it especially helpful for those suffering with low mood and depression.

Lion's mane (*hericium erinaceus*)

So called due to its extraordinarily shaggy 'mane' or long, pale, creamy tendrils, lion's mane reminds me of Dougal, the dog from *The Magic Roundabout* (that dates me) and is perhaps the most powerful of all the easy-to-buy mushrooms when it comes to brain health. Lion's mane has been clinically proven to protect brain cells, guarding against nerve cell damage and neurodegeneration. One of its actions is to stimulate nerve growth factors (NGF), vital for keeping the brain healthy as we age. Supplements can help those with mild dementia and may well play a role in preventing cognitive decline and Alzheimer's. Lion's mane is one of the key supplements I make sure my elderly parents (now in their mid-eighties) take daily. It also improves focus and mental clarity, and I give it to those in my family with attention deficit hyperactivity disorder (ADHD). I also add it to my own coffee, especially when I need to concentrate on a task demanding my full attention and brain power.

Maitake (*grifola frondosa*)

Also known as 'hen of the woods', maitake has the classically, flat, fringed appearance of fungi you sometimes see at the bottom of trees in dark, damp woodlands. An immune-modulator, maitake rose to fame during the Covid-19 pandemic for its ability to stimulate the immune system and increase white blood cell activity, as well as for its naturally high level of vitamin D. Maitake is also a powerful adaptogen (all mushrooms are adaptogenic, meaning they help the body 'adapt' to whatever it needs, be it lifting us up when we need a tonic or calming us down when we feel overwhelmed by stress), with significant antidepressant effects and is helpful for downregulating stress, while supporting the nervous system, making it a good option for combatting feelings of overwhelm.

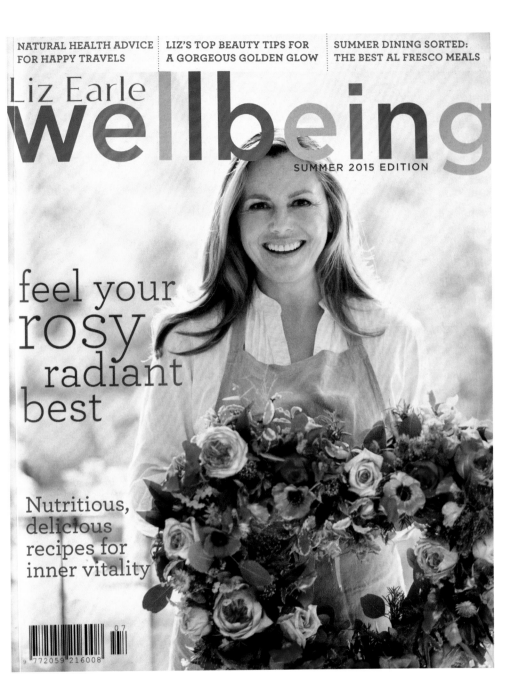

Liz Earle
wellbeing

SUMMER 2015 EDITION

feel your
rosy
radiant
best

Nutritious,
delicious
recipes for
inner vitality

9 772059 216008

The launch of *Liz Earle Wellbeing* magazine – still one of my favourite
covers and my mantra for mid-life women.

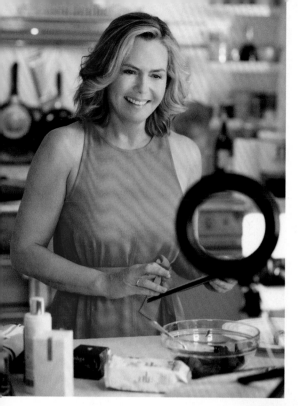

Appearing live on *This Morning* during lockdown meant setting up my laptop in the kitchen to broadcast to the nation! It also encouraged me to start my daily Instagram 'lives', which I still do a couple of times a week now from wherever I happen to be on @LizEarleWellbeing Instagram.

Podcasting is one of my favourite ways of doing a deep-dive into the research. Here recording for the Liz Earle Wellbeing Show podcast in my Wellbeing Studios with Lily in 2020.

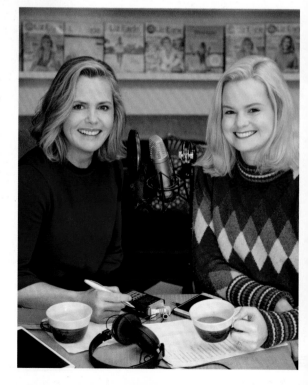

Lift weights to stay strong! I wish I'd picked up my weights sooner as they really are a girl's best friend when it comes to maintaining muscle mass, strength and stamina as we age.

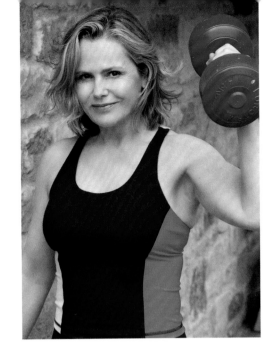

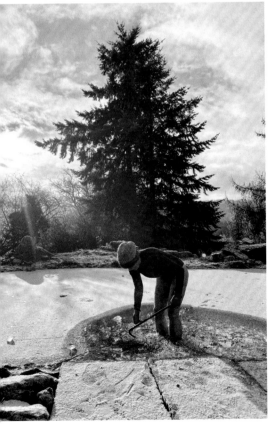

Breaking the ice on the pond in my garden – I had to buy a crowbar! Whether it's a cold shower or a cold dip, 60 seconds of cold exposure is my daily non-negotiable to lift my mood and get the blood circulation going. It's never easy though, especially in winter . . .

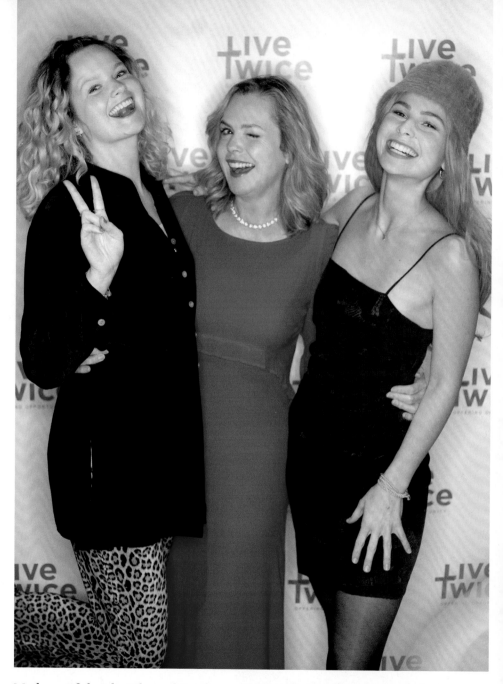

My beautiful girls, Lily and Brella, at my LiveTwice charity's annual Christmas carol concert in 2022. I founded this humanitarian charity back in 2010 as a practical way to give back to those with far less opportunity than I've been fortunate enough to have. I hope this legacy of purpose is something all five of my children will want to continue being involved with in the future too.

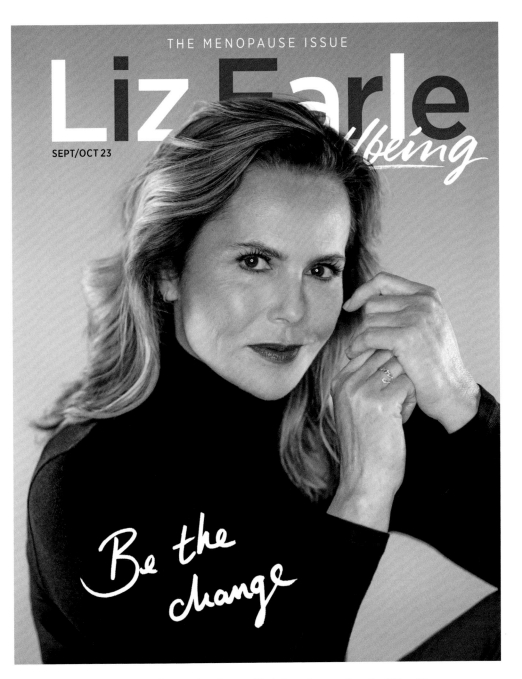

THE MENOPAUSE ISSUE

Liz Earle
Wellbeing

SEPT/OCT 23

Be the change

I'm so proud to have been the first official ambassador for The Menopause Charity and have written several books on the subject. It's been good to raise more awareness of this important life stage and we've achieved a lot in recent years, but there's still so much more to do.

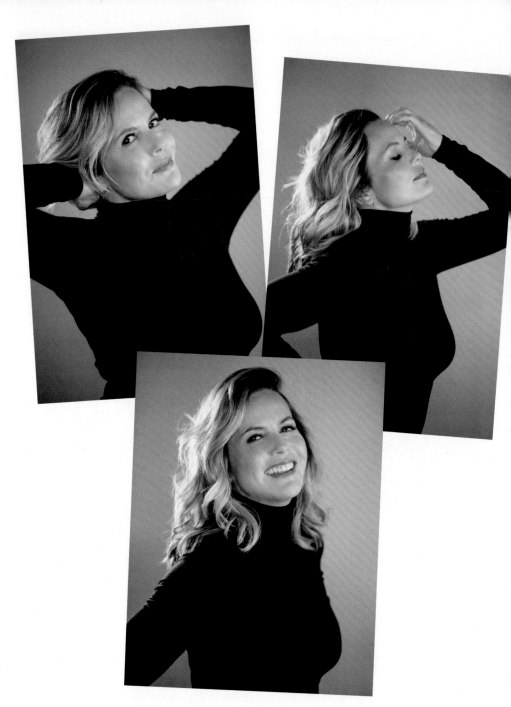

We dedicated an entire magazine issue to topics around the perimenopause and menopause – these are some of my favourite images that didn't make it onto the cover.

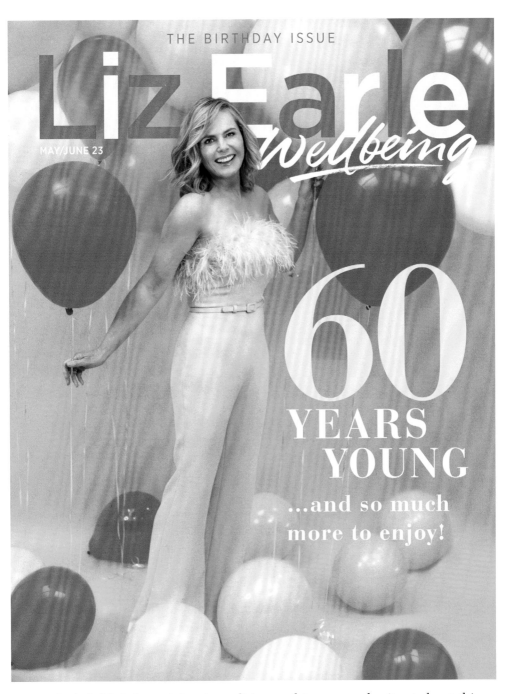

Liz Earle *wellbeing*

MAY/JUNE 23

60
YEARS
YOUNG
...and so much
more to enjoy!

My sixtieth birthday celebration edition and I was *very* hesitant about this cover. My initial reaction to the idea was 'no way!', as I felt embarrassed by my age and just wanted to hide it. But my team persuaded me to go loud and proud – and I'm glad we did as the reaction was so positive!

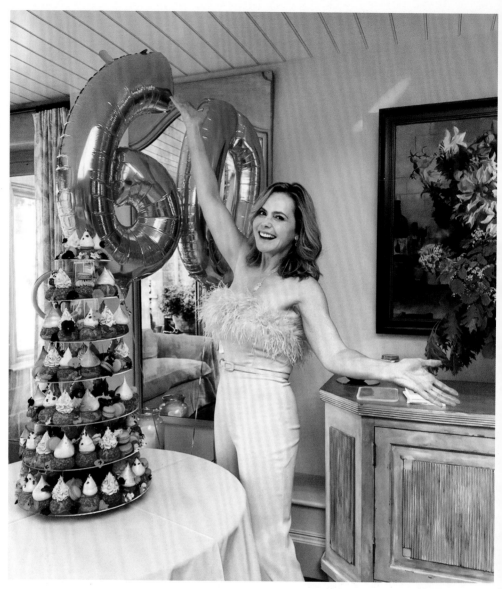

Smashing the taboo of ageism on my Instagram with this post from my birthday celebrations. Having been fearful of wearing a tight pink marabou jumpsuit for my magazine shoot, I ended up buying it to wear at my birthday party here.

Reishi (*ganoderma lucidum*)

Also known as the 'mushroom of spiritual potency' there are many reasons to love reishi. With its powerful anti-inflammatory and immune-supporting properties, reishi is also a powerful adaptogen. Clinical trials have proved its powers at regulating the nervous system, with both a neuroprotective and antidepressant effect. Research into reishi reveals it can also support the endocrine (hormone) system, soothing overactive adrenals and promoting a feeling of peaceful calm.

Shiitake (*lentinula edodes*)

One of the few functional mushrooms to be found on some supermarket shelves, fresh or dried, to use in recipes for their rich, savoury taste, these are extraordinarily abundant in beta-glucans (see page 230) and vitamin D. A popular anti-cancer treatment in TCM, shiitake forms part of the complementary therapy for some cancer patients in Far East Asia today. Shiitake also contains kojic acid, a natural skin brightener used in some acne treatments. Powerfully anti-inflammatory, shiitake have been proven to support the immune system and those who trialled shiitake's isolated active component showed a statistically significant improvement to their mental health in terms of mood and feelings of wellbeing.

Turkey tail (*trametes versicolor*)

One of the most highly researched for its anti-cancer properties, this mushroom gets its name from its colourful stripes and fan-like shape. It contains two unique compounds, polysaccharopeptide (PSP) and polysaccharide-K (PSK), used in Japan for a variety of cancer treatments, including for gastric cancer. Also associated with better lung health, turkey tail can help support the respiratory system, as well as autoimmune diseases and better gut health. Animal studies show the extract enabled them to exercise for longer without becoming tired and, as far as the brain is concerned, turkey tail has been linked to improved memory and even better brain function.

The more I get to know our fungal friends, the more I love them. But – never forage for your own unless you are absolutely sure you know what you're doing! Many mushrooms look the same and some are deadly. Always be guided by a trusted and experienced expert here. I find the easiest way to use mushrooms therapeutically is by adding a splash of tincture to warm drinks. They obviously have a mushroomy flavour; shiitake is a umami – a food flavour enhancer, like monosodium glutamate (MSG) – but without the negative reaction some can experience, so can enhance the taste of hot drinks. Reishi tastes quite bitter, but I find all mushroom tinctures, including reishi, work well in coffee or cocoa. They're also good when added as flavours to soups, sauces and dressings, so my bottles of medicinal mushrooms live in the kitchen, between the cooker and the coffee machine, reminding me to use them often.

Brain Gym

Neuroscientists used to think the brain was static and simply degenerated with age. We now know about neuroplasticity, the ability to grow new brain cells, rewire, restructure and expand areas of the brain previously thought to be beyond repair. One of the easiest and most effective ways to improve brain plastic-ity is to learn a new activity, especially one that involves a differ-ent set of skills. For example, if you're a keen chess player, take up a ball and racquet sport – or vice versa. Crosswords, puzzles and word games are also good, but should be balanced with something involving motor skills and hand–eye coordination. Those of us forever trying to get our kids off their screens or to put down their gaming consoles may be surprised to hear that video games can be good news for the brain. Gaming requires concentration, coordination, speedy reaction times, memory and spatial navigation, which are all useful brain skills. Especially for us older folk, this may mean learning new dexterity skills and even a whole new language of acronyms and gamer chat. 3D adventure games help with memory, problem-solving and picture recognition, while puzzles support brain connectivity and spatial prediction (Sudoku is especially good for this). These days, instead of kicking my kids off their gaming, I'm more likely to ask if I can join in.

Learning a new language is also a powerful brain tool. A study of native English-speaking exchange students studying in Germany found the grey matter in their brains increased after five months of language study, and further studies confirm we can get the same benefit when older too. Music helps improve focus and concentra-tion with studies showing we get greater memory recall when background music is playing while we're reading. Learning a musi-cal instrument brings even greater benefits, as do travel and being exposed to new sights, sounds and experiences – a great excuse for a brain-healthy getaway or two. Getting creative with drawing and painting also improves cognitive function. I enjoy some of the free online tutorials on YouTube that teach you how to draw, from a simple cartoon character to leave on a note for my youngest to a botanical illustration to better know a plant I'm researching or planting in the garden.

> **Doodling is good for the brain, as a bit of mindless pencil flow allows it to switch off from 'action' mode and unfocus, leading to more mindfulness and relaxation.**

Meditation Matters

When it comes to switching off and allowing the brain to rest and recharge, it's hard to find a more effective method than meditation. I learnt the art of Vedic meditation from Jillian Lavender, a wonderful teacher and co-founder of the London Meditation Centre, after I interviewed her for my podcast show. I was fascinated by the way she explained the science of how meditation works to not only relieve stress, but also recharge and repair damaged brains. Meditation is not mindfulness, because mindfulness involves effort to focus, for example on the beauty of a tree or object – not a bad thing in itself, but still using brain energy and thoughts to concentrate on being actively present or 'mindful' in the moment. Meditation is different, in that the mind settles into a non-thinking state, allowing both brain and body to fully rest. Mindfulness is actually an outcome of meditation, as once you come out of a meditative state, you automatically find yourself more aware and present in the moment. Vedic meditation is an offshoot of Transcendental Meditation, or TM, popularised by The Beatles back in 1968 when they famously went to Rishikesh in India to hang out with Maharishi

Mahesh Yogi. TM has been the subject of hundreds of scientific studies showing its wide-ranging benefits for body and brain. Specifically, it's been shown to thicken the prefrontal cortex, the part of the brain that manages 'higher order function' such as decision-making and concentration. Fascinating neuroimaging has also shown that regular meditation helps prevent age-related brain shrinkage. It also significantly lowers the stress hormone cortisol while increasing levels of brain-derived neurotrophic factor (BDNF), improving memory and general brain power.

Both Vedic meditation and TM use a mantra, a word that has no meaning, which you repeat silently over and over again in your head as you sink into a deeper state of wakeful relaxation. You sit upright (so as not to fall asleep!), close your eyes and focus on the mantra, which gives the brain something mindless to chew on, so it doesn't get distracted by what's on your to-do list. Of course, thoughts do float into your head, but the idea is to simply override them by repeating the mantra. You don't have to stop thinking in order to meditate; in fact, the flow of thoughts is entirely natural and not a sign of failure. You simply allow the mantra to take over and this gradually leads the mind to dive ever deeper towards its innermost layers. Mantras are secret, personally passed on by an experienced instructor and you're told not to write them down or share them with anyone else. I was given my first mantra by a TM instructor 30 years ago when I first wrote about meditation, but I didn't stay with the practice as 'life' overtook me. It was only after meeting Jillian (who later confirmed my mantra was correct for me – as my instructor, she's the only other person I have ever shared it with) that my interest was reignited. Once learnt, you are supposed to practise this form of meditation for 20 minutes twice a day – ideally first thing in the morning and then again at the end of the day (but not just before bed, when you're likely to drift off to sleep). This doesn't always happen for me, but I do feel better for it when it does. And for those who say they're too busy and don't have the time to meditate, I would say, you don't have the time *not* to meditate, as regular meditation actually makes you more productive. Easy wins such as turning off the TV ten minutes earlier or setting your morning alarm ever so slightly earlier to get this done really do make a positive difference.

Brain-Boosting Moves

Last but not least, movement matters. Just as we can physically work the body, so we can also work the brain. A multitude of studies link physical activity with improved brain capacity, and not just the aerobic kind that increases oxygen capacity to boost blood supply to the top of the head. Of course, moving the body circulates fresh oxygen around the brain, improving blood flow and the delivery of brain-enhancing nutrients, but studies show that slow movement, such as walking and tai chi, also boost the number of new nerve cells in the brain and increase the proteins that help these neurons thrive.

Yoga and Pilates are especially beneficial for the brain, as any kind of inversion (think downward-facing dog or headstands) stimulates the pituitary gland, increasing the cerebrospinal fluid of the central nervous system. According to Assistant Professor of Neuropsychology at the University of California, San Francisco Memory and Aging Center, Kaitlin Casaletto, 'this is where the magic happens when it comes to cognition', as any form of physical activity keeps brain synapses (small pockets of space between neurons) healthy, enabling them to communicate better. This is good news for any more sedentary folk who may balk at the thought of taking up some kind of strenuous activity in the second half of life. Her studies of participants (average age 70) show it's never too late to start, and in her words 'you don't have to be a gym rat either'.

Of course, vigorous activity is a good option and regular aerobic exercise is directly correlated to the size of the hippocampus, the part of the brain controlling learning and verbal recall. MRI scans of more than 2,000 people aged 60 or over showed the more active they were, the larger their hippocampus. But in even better news, the protective effects were highest in those over the age of 75. Even six to seven minutes of vigorous activity sees an improvement in cognition and memory function. Lifting weights (which I'll come on to in more detail in the next chapter) appears to be especially beneficial for the brain as well as the body, as it focuses the mind on performing specific movements, which, in turn, gives our neural circuits a good workout too. Moving the body can also be sociable and fun, with a study of elderly people showing that regular dancing reduced the risk of dementia by 76 per cent – twice as much as reading.

Switching off our brains

The brain needs good quality sleep in order to rest and repair. Sleep is when our brains have time to catch up on their house-keeping, processing memories and activities from the day. It needs time to tidy up and file the paperwork. In terms of brain health as we age, the impact of getting a good night's sleep cannot be overestimated, especially when it comes to lowering anxiety levels and dampening down stress responses. I'll share ways to get a better night's sleep in Chapter 10.

Our brains are mostly made of fats and so need a steady supply of healthy fats to support them, especially as we age. Make sure you include plenty of good quality fats in your daily diet – yet another compelling reason why midlife is not the time to go low-fat. Don't over-look the importance of sleep for better brain health, move more and consider twice-daily meditation. Taking time out is not lazy, it's a proac-tive part of cognition and mental clarity, which gives you more time to do things better.

Healthy hacks
- Add in a daily dose of fish oils, specifically DHA from fish oil or krill supplements.
- Consider adding in one or two brain-boosting botanicals such as ginkgo biloba and step into the magical world of mushrooms (notably lion's mane in this context).
- Learn a new skill, especially one that is outside your norm, and find a new way to move, such as yoga, Pilates or tai chi. It doesn't have to be strenuous. And take up meditation, a new skill in itself.

CHAPTER 9

Movement Matters

The thing I've learnt about exercise in midlife is that it doesn't have to be for long and it doesn't have to be complicated – it just has to happen! I've learnt so much from leading personal trainer Michael Garry, a valued contributor to Liz Earle Wellbeing magazine and website, where you can find many of his videos training me. He says that, when it comes to exercise, consistency matters more than time. Squeezing in just ten minutes of simple squats, lunges, push-ups and stretches each day can be more valuable and beneficial in the long term than a weekend high-intensity gym session or lengthy park run. This is good news as, let's be real here, we can all find ten minutes in the morning before a busy day gets hold of us.

If you can get some exercise outdoors first thing in the morning, you're doing yourself a real favour. As I explained earlier, early-morning light has the most powerful effect when it comes to setting up our circadian rhythm, energising brain and body first thing and setting up your internal body clock for the rest of the day (see page 259).

Physical activity guidelines

The official recommended guidance for an adult to maintain good health is to do the following:

- At least 150 minutes of moderate aerobic activity such as cycling or brisk walking every week, and
- strength exercises on two or more days a week that work all the major muscles (legs, hips, back, abdomen, chest, shoulders and arms).

Or:

- 75 minutes of vigorous aerobic activity such as running or a game of singles tennis every week, and
- strength exercises on two or more days a week that work all the major muscles (legs, hips, back, abdomen, chest, shoulders and arms).

Or:

- A mix of moderate and vigorous aerobic activity every week – for example, 2 x 30-minute runs plus 30 minutes of brisk walking equates to 150 minutes of moderate aerobic activity, and
- strength exercises on two or more days a week that work all the major muscles (legs, hips, back, abdomen, chest, shoulders and arms).

A good rule is that one minute of vigorous activity provides the same health benefits as two minutes of moderate activity. One way to do your recommended 150 minutes of weekly physical activity is to do 30 minutes on 5 days every week.

All adults should also break up long periods of sitting with light activity. Set an alarm or timer on your phone to get up from your chair and move (even just a walk around the room) once an hour.

*Source: **NHS website***

How to Start Running in Midlife

I've lost count of the number of my friends who reach midlife, often a milestone birthday such as 40, 50 or even beyond, and announce that they're going to run a marathon. My reaction is usually to try to dissuade them – why? Because running beyond a certain amount of time/distance is actually counterproductive as it lowers the immune system and can have a negative effect on our bone strength (as well as lead to injury and a lengthy recovery time). So how far is too far when it comes to running? According to Michael Garry, anything over 5k can start to have negative effects. He says running 5k is the perfect distance for stamina and strength, without triggering an adverse immune response. Having cracked the 5k target, if you want to up your game, simply speed up your time. Not only does this make you more agile and lighter on your feet, but it also revs up the metabolism so you burn fat faster and makes you more dynamic.

I will make a confession to you here: I came to running late in life. I was in my late forties when I started training with Michael, in an attempt to shift the baby weight that had stubbornly settled around my middle (which I now know was triggered by my perimenopause). I remember looking at my middle-aged shape in the mirror and thinking, I really don't want to be fat and 50 – triggered by vanity, but also in the knowledge that if I didn't get a grip and address my fitness, I might never do it. Being more active (specifically with aerobic exercise) is also increasingly being linked to longevity, as it stimulates our stem cells to generate new bone and muscle mass. The first time I met Michael, I asked for some guidance and help getting back in shape, quickly adding, 'but, I DON'T RUN'. In fact, I had never run, not even a jog. I just felt that it wasn't for me and, frankly, I couldn't understand my keen-bean friends who'd slip into a pair of trainers wherever in the world they happened to be at the time.

Fast-forward a decade or so, and I now absolutely love running! OK, so I don't do it for very long or go very far (or very fast) – I will never be a race-runner – but I do love everything about it: the powerful surge of happy endorphins released after the first five minutes or so, the feel of fabulously fresh air against my skin and the fact that my brain gets the chance to disconnect from the day-to-day and can be free. Many of my best ideas happen during a run and I always, without fail, feel physically, mentally and emotionally better for it. During lockdown, I invested in a second-hand running machine, but actually prefer the great outdoors, with its added benefit of feeling part of the elements (yes, I do run in the rain – it feels wonderfully freeing) and the chance to connect with a more natural world, even if it's a city park and not my rural West Country home turf.

Never say never and be open to the possibilities of running.

Start small: alternate between a one-minute walk and a two-minute jog, building up slowly and enjoying the satisfaction of clocking your progress, day by day, week by week. Run with a friend if you fancy the company or need the incentive – and use the 'Couch to 5k' app as a helpful running guide (see page 306). I've also invested in a simple under-desk treadmill and use this to avoid sitting at my desk for long periods of time. It fits neatly under a standing desk and you simply stand on it as you work, walking either on the flat or on a slight incline as you do your desk job. It takes a bit of getting used to (Zoom calls are a little disconcerting as you're moving as you speak!), but it's such an easy, sneaky exercise habit and I find myself walking for miles without even thinking about it – perfect for getting in those 10,000 steps a day while you're working; the ultimate in multitasking efficiency.

My Ten-Minute Guide to Midlife Fitness

Talk to any professional fitness trainer and they'll inevitably highlight the same few exercises as their go-tos when it comes to teaching clients. These are some of the ones I highlighted in my morning routine on page 37. Each one is simple to do wherever you happen to be, doesn't need any special equipment and relies mostly on your own body weight as a form of resistance. Each activates and strengthens important muscle groups, helps burn fat and builds a stronger, firmer and more toned physique. You'll find illlustrations to accompany each of these moves here: lizearlewellbeing.com/bshlinks.

Lunges

These can either be static lunges on the spot or a walking lunge. The aim is to step forward on alternate legs, lowering the front knee to create a 45-degree angle before standing up again and repeating on the other side. You can hold weights as you get stronger. I do sets of 20 on each side, and have even moved on to one-legged squats, resting one leg behind me on a bench or chair. This is great for stability – just be sure to have something to grab hold of should you start to topple over.

Walking lunges are easy to do outside (or in a largeish room). Admittedly, doing these outside does make you look like John Cleese in the Ministry of Funny Walks sketch from Monty Python, but they are a good inclusion into your daily stroll. Keep arms raised straight above the head for maximum benefit.

Benefits: lunges strengthen the lower body muscles including your core, so be sure to pull your tummy in as you lunge. This exercise also improves balance and increases hip flexibility.

Squats

Stand with your feet shoulder-width apart, knees over your middle toes. Lower your backside by hinging at the hips and bending the knees, keeping them over your middle toes and heels on the ground. Keep your head and chest upright, eyes looking forward. Repeat!

You can squat with or without weights. I started without before introducing and then gradually increasing my weights to around an 18kg kettlebell in each hand. I do these in sets of 25 at a time.

Not only will doing squats give you a perkier backside and more shapely calves, they're also a super-fast way to speed the metabolism and burn fat. Weighted squats activate every major muscle group in the body and work out the abdominals too. Squats of every kind are what's known as a functional exercise, especially important as we age. We all want to be able to get out of a chair easily or bend down to pick up something from the bottom shelf of the grocery store with ease. Studies show that our ability to sit and rise from the floor is even a good prediction of living longer.

If you find holding heavy weights uncomfortable, slip on a weighted vest or jacket. This spreads additional weight across your upper back, working the shoulder muscles as well as adding additional weights for the glutes.

Benefits: the more muscles we use, the more calories we burn, so squats are a great flab-fighter. Daily squats should form part of your everyday routine. There's no excuse not to do a few squats daily – try doing them while brushing your teeth. Studies show that squats are even good for the brain, as the down–up movement sends neurological signals that are vital for building new, healthy brain cells, improving cognition and critical thinking, especially as we get older.

Press-ups

If you're new to press-ups and unsure about how to start, begin with a simple standing version with hands flat against a wall and push yourself forward and back. You can then move to doing press-ups on your knees, remembering to keep your navel pulled in towards the spine. As you get stronger, you can move on to full-body press-ups, balancing on your toes, heels pushed back and body perpendicular to the floor. As with squats, the down–up movement here also specifically improves brain power. I do sets of 30 full-body press-ups, aiming for at least 60 repetitions.

As you progress, you can make your press-ups even harder by bringing your hands much closer together. Lower your body as before, until your elbows are behind you at a 90-degree angle. Sounds easy? Try it – it's a killer!

Benefits: a full press-up fires up just about every major muscle group in the body and is an aerobic activity, flooding your cells with fresh oxygen and releasing endorphins in the brain, so you feel happier as well as stronger. The more you do, the easier they become. One study found that those who can do full press-ups are 96 per cent less likely to experience a cardiovascular problem in later life.

Tricep dips

This is another excellent resistance exercise using your own body weight to strengthen and tone the shoulders, triceps, upper back and chest. You'll need a bench or sturdy chair to grip hold of behind you as you lower your bottom to the floor and back up again. Stretch one foot out in front of you for even more of a workout and to improve balance.

Tricep dips are also great for the abdominals, so don't forget to engage your core before you start. Dips also strengthen your grip and the 'grip test' is a reliable indicator of how well you're ageing. As a general rule, those with the strongest hands tend to be strong elsewhere, so this simple test is often used by doctors to assess overall strength. Medics will use a dynamometer to measure how hard and how long you can maintain a good squeeze, but you can get a good indication of your strength at home by seeing how long you can grip-hold a heavy object, such as a bag of potatoes held out in front of you.

Once you've mastered the basic tricep dip technique, you can move on to doing forward-facing dips from a set of bars. I've treated myself to a set of bars at home, which I found very hard to use at first, but have worked up to doing a few sets of ten at a time. I'm working towards managing a full-body pull-up, but that's a goal I have yet to achieve. This exercise not only needs a great deal of strength but also a low amount of body fat, as the heavier you are, the more weight you have to pull up . . .

Benefits: considered the best exercise for toning and strengthening muscles in the triceps (the muscle on the backs of your arms) and will quickly build arm and shoulder strength, as well as blast away flabby upper arm 'bingo wings'.

Crunches

Lie on your back with your knees bent at 90 degrees, feet crossed at the ankles to protect your back. Support your head with your hands with elbows pointing outwards and pull your navel in towards your spine. Lift your head, neck and shoulders away from the floor, taking care not to pull on your neck. Slowly lower and repeat. I aim to do sets of 50 at a time. You can also incorporate a side twist as you lift, touching your elbow to the opposite knee, to work the oblique muscles on either side of the abdomen.

Crunches are far more effective than full sit-ups as our primary abdominal muscles are only activated during the first 30–45 degrees of movement, so doing a full sit-up is a waste of time and effort. However, they're not always necessary as heavily weighted squats will also firm the abs and strengthen your core.

Benefits: crunches support your core or middle section of the body, encourage better posture and make it easier (and safer) to lift heavy objects without damaging your back. They'll also help shrink the waist and give the abdomen a nice bit of definition.

A word about the pelvic floor

We're probably all aware of the importance of strengthening the pelvic floor, the 'sling' of muscle fibres that supports important parts of the lower body (including the bladder and rectum), as well as those that are specifically female (the uterus, cervix and vagina). We lose pelvic floor strength as we age, partly due to the general loss of collagen and connective tissue, but also as we lose oestrogen that supports these (another reason why HRT is so helpful for health as we age – see pages 92–94). Strengthening the pelvic floor also helps prevent pelvic organ prolapse, a common issue for women in midlife and beyond. This is when the pelvic floor weakens or becomes loose (for example, after childbirth) and allows the pelvic organs to drop down and press into, or even out of, the vagina. Prolapse is treatable and the sooner it is addressed the easier it is to rectify, so do speak to your doctor if you suspect this might be an issue (if you feel a heaviness in the vagina or experience any kind of incontinence, for example).

Doing pelvic floor exercises – squeezing the internal muscles inside the vagina and around the rectum and holding for a count of ten before releasing – is something we should all be doing on a daily basis, ideally at least three times a day. You'll find plenty of specific free expert guidance on this from women's health physios online.

How to Get Started with Weights

Taking up weight-lifting might not be the first thing that springs to mind when considering ways to work out in midlife, but trust me, a set of dumbbells can be your new best friend. Lifting weights, such as simple dumbbells or kettlebells, not the circus-style strong-man iron bars, is one of the very best ways for women to preserve muscle mass as they age. Using any kind of weight (a dumbbell or your own body weight) for exercise builds muscle tone and definition, without giving you the shape of a bodybuilder. For the average woman, lifting a few weights strengthens joints, prevents muscle loss and builds better bone health.

**Feeling strong is a powerful and
priceless confidence booster.**

Truth be told, if we don't lift weights, we'll age faster. Sarcopenia, or muscle loss, happens at the rate of around 1 per cent or more each year after the age of 30. Loss of oestrogen during perimenopause and beyond accelerates this loss, also reducing bone density and making us more likely to develop osteoporosis and bone fractures. Losing our muscle strength obviously leaves us weaker as we age, more likely to suffer a physical injury as well as worse metabolic health. With physical weakness comes a real feeling of getting old, of not being able to do the things we'd like to do, having less energy and motivation to embrace and enjoy life to the full. Weight-lifting can help reverse this trend. This is due to putting our bones under weight-bearing stress, forcing them to grow stronger and increase in density in order to cope. Building up our muscle mass also protects against weight gain, as the more lean muscle tissue we have, the faster the rate at which we burn energy. Skeletal muscle is a metabolically active tissue, burning dietary carbs and body fat to fuel the body's daily activities. The more muscle, the higher our basal metabolic rate, resulting in a greater number of calories burnt over a day, meaning we can eat more without piling on the pounds. This is especially significant as we age, a time when our basal metabolic rate drops (one reason why middle-age spread occurs).

If you've never picked up a weight before, it is worth getting some personal guidance. Most gyms will offer a free introductory session and there are also a huge number of beginner tutorials on YouTube showing exactly how to do weighted exercises with the correct form to minimise risk of injury. Start small and slow – but do start.

Resistance bands are easy and inexpensive and can be used for leg and arm workouts using varying degrees of tension (the stronger the band, the greater the resistance as the harder it is to pull apart). Once your muscle fibres are used to a bit of regular activation, move on up to dumbbells. Start with a weight that you can lift 10–15 times under control without losing your posture. Begin with one or two sets of 10–15 repetitions, resting for 60 seconds between each set. I have two sets of weights under my bed, a pair of 6kg dumbbells that I use for bicep curls and front-arm raises, plus a pair of much heavier 18kg kettlebell weights that I use when I do my squats (often still wearing my pyjamas). I started with much lighter weights though, and have gradually moved on up the scale. Be patient with your progress and it's important to give your body a day or two of rest between sessions for muscles to recover. And don't forget to stretch after each session too.

When it comes to longevity, one of the most exciting discoveries regarding weightlifting in later life is research showing it encourages the growth of new muscle and bone stem cells. This is highly significant, as tissue regeneration declines with age. If something as simple as lifting a few weights can actually reverse this – bring it on! Studies also show that weight-bearing exercise influences stem cells to turn themselves into bone, not fat. So while we might not see a reduction in our overall weight on the scales, we are likely to find our bones become heavier, denser and stronger as our fat reserves dwindle.

Eating a high-protein diet and adding in some resistance movement on a daily basis really are two simple keys to a longer, stronger and more energised life.

Supplements for Strength

You don't have to be a gym bunny to benefit from taking a few supplements to enhance the effects of exercise. I've already mentioned protein powders and these come into their own when we work out as a fast and effective way to provide muscle fibres with the fuel they need to increase and strengthen (see page 137). My all-time favourite supplement for strength, though, is creatine, a natural compound made from the amino acids arginine, glycine and methionine. It's present in meat, fish and dairy products, as well as widely available as a flavourless powder you add to food and drinks. The body makes creatine from animal protein food sources, but its ability to do this declines by around 8 per cent

A BETTER SECOND HALF

every 10 years after the age of 30. Previously the preserve of high-performance athletes, creatine is one of the most studied nutrients. It is genuinely safe and effective, and I think all midlifers should consider taking it every day, regardless of exercise, as it brings so many benefits for preserving muscle strength and brain energy. I do. Having studied the data, I'm now never without it. But don't just take my word for it. The position statement of the International Society of Sports Nutrition on creatine states: 'Creatine monohydrate is the most effective ergonomic nutritional supplement currently available to athletes in terms of increasing high-intensity exercise capacity and lean body mass during training.' In other words, creatine helps us work out harder by boosting ATP energy production in the brain (see page 62), while making us look leaner. What's not to love?

Not only very safe, creatine also helps prevent muscle injury and has more recently been linked with many other protective health benefits due to its immune-regulating properties, helping fibromyalgia, traumatic brain injury, depression and chronic fatigue syndrome. It's even being associated with reducing the risk of developing Parkinson's, Huntington's and Alzheimer's diseases. A study looking at potential benefits for improving memory in the elderly reported that subjects with an average age of 76 saw improvements in long-term memory when given 20g a day of creatine for just one week. A staggering result – and one that has got me buying additional supplies for my own elderly parents. In terms of exercise benefits, just 3–5g (around 1tsp) of creatine powder stirred into a cup of coffee, tea, smoothie, porridge or yoghurt is enough to give our muscles an immediate hit of energy. It's also cheap as well as being highly effective – a win–win.

You can't outrun what's on your plate, but movement and strength training can change your body shape and are crucial for retaining muscle mass and bone density. This is especially significant for midlife and older women, at risk of developing osteoporosis. You don't have to do much, but you do have to do something. Exercise needs to move up the priority list as we age and cannot be an optional extra. If you're unsure where to begin, start by walking. Getting outdoors first thing is an especially good habit, so invest in some all-weather walking shoes and get out there.

Healthy hacks
- Never sit for longer than an hour without taking a break to get up, stretch and walk about, even if only for a few moments. If you work at a desk, consider a standing desk and under-desk walking treadmill.
- Buy a tub of creatine. Add 1tsp to a warm drink (or yoghurt, porridge, kefir or smoothie) and make this a new daily ritual, for both body and brain.
- Treat your body to a set of dumbbells – lighter weights for bicep curls and a heavier set for weighted squats. Keep them somewhere you can see them to remind yourself to lift them often.

CHAPTER 10

Ways to Rest and Recharge

It's tempting to overlook how vital sleep is for our overall health and longevity. It's just collapsing into bed and letting the body do the best it can, right? Wrong. Sleep is one of the most fundamentally *active* aspects of living and ageing well. We can spend a huge amount of time (and money) to eat well, go to the gym, swallow pricey supplements and all the rest, but without a good night's sleep (which is free!) much of that effort will be worthless. We spend around a third of our lives asleep, so let's do it well and reap the longevity benefits.

The Importance of Sleep

Sleep is a continuous cycle of four different stages, each lasting 70–120 minutes, repeating 4–5 times during a 7–9-hour night's sleep. The first three stages are non-REM (rapid eye movement) sleep and the fourth is deep REM sleep.

Stage 1: the initial dropping-off phase as we fall lightly asleep and our brainwaves and heartbeat slow down. This lasts around seven minutes.

Stage 2: moderately light sleep, as our muscles relax throughout the body, heart rate further falls, brainwaves briefly rise then slow back down to a gentle rhythm and body temperature lowers. We spend most of the night in this stage of sleep.

Stage 3: the start of deep sleep. Eyes and muscles stop moving or twitching, brainwaves slow even further and the body sets about its practical repair work, renewing cells, proteins, muscle fibres and more.

Stage 4: REM sleep, the deepest stage. We arrive here after around 90 minutes of non-REM sleep. At this point, our eyes dart from side to side, brainwaves and heartbeat increase and we breathe more quickly. REM sleep is when we dream and it's also the point when the brain processes information from the day, crucial for making memories and learning from experience. A healthy brain needs several cycles of deep REM sleep each night.

It's also important to note that sleep follows these clearly defined cycles, which is why uninterrupted sleep is so important (not having to get up for a wee, to soothe a crying child or to let the dog out). REM cycles are especially important.

The process of sleep activates many unique and important biological processes. While the body is resting and the mind doesn't have to focus on getting 'stuff' done, the brain uses this 'downtime' to clear out the trash, get rid of the toxic waste that gets built up around cells, re-organise neurological pathways, recharge gut microbes, repair damaged tissues, synthesise proteins and release important hormones. When it comes to ageing, one of the most important aspects of sleep is activating the brain's glymphatic (waste disposal) system, which sweeps away toxic by-products produced by cellular activity in the brain, so we wake feeling more refreshed and well. A good night's sleep also improves memory function, because during deep sleep our brains convert short-term memories of the day into long-term memories to recall in the future.

Several specific areas of our brains actually become more active after we've had the chance to sleep, including the amygdala (the area that regulates emotions and how we feel), the hippocampus (controlling memory) and the medial prefrontal cortex (which controls attention span and ability to think clearly). Our immune systems depend on a good night's sleep too, as we make antibodies and immune cells while we sleep. If we don't get enough sleep, insufficient antibodies may be made, making us more susceptible to viruses and disease.

Sleep is also linked to our digestion: the better our sleep, the broader the diversity of beneficial microbes in our guts. Researchers at the American Gut Project studying over 10,000 participants have also found that better sleep increases the ratio of a relatively newly discovered bacterium called *Akkermansia*, the so-called 'anti-fat bug' linked to a reduced risk of obesity. In studies, those with the highest levels of this bacterium correspondingly have the lowest levels of body fat. Sleep also influences weight control in other ways, regulating the hormones that influence when, and how much, we eat. These include ghrelin, which increases appetite, and leptin, which increases satiety or the feeling of fullness after eating. Lack of sleep causes ghre-lin to rise, so we're more likely to reach for that family-sized crisp packet, whereas good quality sleep produces more leptin, quelling the urge to snack.

Sleep well

Unfortunately, it would seem that despite a growing awareness of its benefits, more of us are finding it harder to get good quality sleep. A study by the healthcare charity Nuffield Health shows that soaring numbers of us are suffering with insomnia. In fact, this 2020 study showed that the majority of us are having a worse night's sleep when compared to the previous year. Staggeringly, researchers found that out of the 8,000 adults surveyed, 1 in 10 people were getting only 2–4 hours' sleep per night, with younger adults getting the least sleep overall. This is deeply worrying. Just one night's poor sleep can affect mood, concentration and capabilities the following day, with long-term sleep disruptions triggering negative thinking, anxiety and depression. So if poor sleep is something you've grown to accept, it's time to take some action.

Setting your circadian rhythm

We all have an unconscious internal body clock – our circadian clock – that regulates the daily cycle of sleep and wakefulness, hunger, hormones, digestion and more besides. The circadian clock is basically a clump of neurons called the suprachiasmatic nucleus (SCN), found in the hypothalamus at the base of the brain. When our eyes sense daylight, they activate signals that stimulate the SCN, telling the brain it's time to wake up. The SCN then releases a series of hormones, including the stress hormone cortisol, to activate the body and get us mobilised for the day. Light is the most important factor here; even when our eyes are closed, they still sense the light and activate these wake-up signals. When the sun rises, the body starts to produce cortisol to stir us. Then, as the day progresses and we start to feel tired, the pineal gland in the brain releases melatonin, a hormone that influences when, and how well, we sleep. This natural ebb and flow of daylight and its effect on our hormones is known as the circadian rhythm.

Circadian rhythm is guided by natural events in the environment around us – like daylight – but it can be altered by other factors, such as meal times and genetics. These are 'set' over our lifetime and can be hard, but not impossible, to change. Some of us will have a genetic disposition to rise early (the larks), while others, like myself, are night owls, preferring to get more of our activities done later in the day. It is possible to retrain the body to want to get up earlier (see page 261 for my tips on this). Eating late in the evening also disrupts the circadian rhythm, as the process of digestion and changes in body temperature that happen around this interfere with sleep (one reason why late-night eating is not a good idea). Circadian rhythm also shifts with age. Teenagers are notorious for wanting to lie in late, while in older age we find we tend to wake up earlier and want to hit the pillow sooner.

Exercise helps establish a healthy sleep–wake cycle, although it is a stimulant, which is why it is best done in the morning. Caffeine also artificially wakes us up, which is why it's so popular as a drink in the morning, but keep in mind it stays in the system for around six to seven hours in most of us (longer for some), so really should be kept as a morning-only drink, unless you need to stay awake. As well as shift work, jet lag is also a major circadian clock disruptor, so plan your travel days accordingly when crossing significant time zones.

How to get up early

This is a huge life hack. Confession time: I am not an early riser, but little by little I've learnt to get up earlier. How? By setting my alarm ten minutes earlier each week. The more often we do something, the more it becomes a habit. One benefit of growing older is that your internal clock also tends to reset itself to rising earlier. Of course, this needs to be balanced with getting to bed earlier too. I've matched my earlier starts to the day with bringing supper time forward and I choose to eat earlier now than I used to, given the chance. I now greatly enjoy my early mornings when the house is quiet, giving me the chance to 'sort my stuff', do my household chores and make more time for meditation, journaling or watching the sun rise with a steaming mug of tea. An early start also gives you the chance to plan your day, instead of bumbling headlong in a rush to get up. It really is one of the best gifts you can give yourself.

Sleep Problems Solved

Problem: **stress and anxiety** are major factors when it comes to poor sleep and are top of the leader board as reasons we report a bad night in bed. The stress that can build up from pressures during the day increases your heart rate, leading to your mind racing. Your brain then becomes stimulated and you're just too alert to sleep.

Solution: it's easy to say don't stress so much, but that's not always straightforward. A better solution, while you're sorting things through, is to find ways to manage your stress to help you sleep better. Meditation, relaxation and breathing techniques done at any time of the day will help, but especially if just before bed. Emptying your mind before turning off the lights is a good habit. Because your brain uses sleep to do its admin work for the day, you can give it a helping hand by writing down the things that are preying on your mind. Include any crucial bits of information you need to remember in the morning, as offloading these thoughts onto a piece of paper reassures the brain that it no longer needs to keep hold of them, leaving the mind calmer and clearer as it prepares your body to switch off. As well as writing down anything troubling, it's also helpful to make a note of goals for the new day ahead. End your jottings on a positive note. Write down three things (or more) that you're grateful for that day.

Problem: **what and when we eat and drink** can have a huge impact on the quality of our sleep. Eating a carb-heavy meal in the evening, especially one high in refined sugars, causes insulin spikes and surges which the body then has to work hard to digest properly, instead of using that time to restore the rest of the body.

Solution: make sure you finish your last mouthful of food and drink (other than plain water or herb teas) at least two hours before your head hits the pillow.

Problem: **caffeine** is another culprit when it comes to sleep distur-bances. As discussed on page 50, genetics play a large part in whether or not we have a fast response to caffeine and can process it swiftly out of the system. But even those who are fast processors and say 'I can drink espresso after dinner, it has no effect on me' are fooling themselves. Caffeine is a psychoactive stimulant, delaying our falling-asleep mechanism as well as reducing the quality of deep REM sleep.

Solution: those who don't process coffee well (or strong tea, cola/energy drinks or dark chocolate, all containing caffeine) should have their final caffeine fix no later than midday, as it takes 6–12 hours to process it out of the system. No matter what your conscious mind tells you, that late-night espresso or slice of dark chocolate truffle cake is truly best saved for the next day.

**Caffeine leaves a legacy in the brain,
even if we're not aware of it.**

Problem: **I just don't feel tired!** How often have you found your-self lying awake unable to drift off, wondering why it is your body and brain refuse to allow you to sleep? External factors are often the cause, such as the blue light emitted from your small screens.

Solution: don't check emails before bed. It's bad for your brain to receive blue light from a screen as well as start to problem-solve or process communications. Keep your bedroom a device-free zone, leaving all phones, tablets and laptops outside the door. Keep a landline for emergencies and buy an alarm clock (worked perfectly well in the old days). Take a book to bed and read from the printed page and not the glare of an e-reader. Ideally, install old-fashioned halogen or use specific 'dark' lightbulbs (modern LEDs disrupt brainwaves) and/or wear blue light blocking glasses for a couple of hours before bed.

Sleep-Supporting Supplements

If you're still struggling to sleep, these supplements can help:

Magnesium

Our bodies use this electrolyte for hundreds of essential processes, especially within the nervous system, which largely regulates our sleep. Studies show that taking this mighty mineral before bed can improve quality of sleep and help with insomnia, muscle spasms and the restless legs syndrome that can often wake us up in the night. Magnesium also plays a role in maintaining melatonin. Magnesium can be found in many forms and all are likely to be effective, but the one with the most evidence for relaxation is magnesium glycinate, which is the one I take every night before bed. Some supplements specifically promoted for sleep are blended with other soporific ingredients, such as L-theanine, zinc, ashwagandha and DHEA (a hormonal precursor to making melanin that increases during the REM sleep cycle).

L-theanine

This amino acid is a natural relaxant, reported to help us fall asleep more quickly. Studies show that when we take it, our quality of sleep improves – not by acting as a sedative, but by encouraging the neurotransmitters that relax the body and reduce anxiety. L-theanine is found in green and black teas, which is why drinking tea can make us feel good (and not too jittery, as it counteracts the caffeine content). Interesting research has found that taking 400mg daily of L-theanine also improves the sleep quality of boys with ADHD.

Montmorency cherry

These fruits are naturally rich in melatonin, but we would need to eat quite a few to reap their benefits (around 25 sweet or 100 sour Montmorency cherries daily). Drinking regular cherry juice is a simpler option, although it may contain more sugar than the naturally sour Montmorecy cherry versions. One study of the elderly showed that drinking tart cherry juice (such as Montmorency) reduced insomnia. Or take an encapsulated or powdered supplement. Taking a Montmorency cherry supplement 30 minutes before bed can help you to feel sleepy earlier.

Sleepy herbs

There are several herbs that have sedative properties, notably Passiflora, lavender, chamomile and valerian. Passiflora (from the passionflower) has been shown to increase GABA, a calming neurotransmitter, making it especially useful for times when we're feeling anxious and need to switch off our brains for better sleep. Studies trialling Passiflora have found it to be helpful for relieving menopausal symptoms too. Lavender is the scent that helps me drift off to sleep at night and sprinkling a few drops of the oil on my pillow is part of my nightly go-to sleep ritual. Taking lavender supplements, such as tinctures, also show benefits for those with disturbed sleep patterns and general anxiety. Similar studies using chamomile capsules also showed significant benefits when it comes to improved quality of sleep, suggesting a bedtime cup of chamomile could also be beneficial (see page 198).

CBD

Entire books have been written about the staggering benefits to be had from using a good quality CBD oil, but one of the most cited is its power to encourage a better night's sleep. CBD stands for cannabidiol, one of the major cannabinoids found in the cannabis plant. Unlike THC, the psychoactive component of cannabis, CBD is legal to use and widely available, usually in the form of drops or edible gummies. Many studies show that CBD has a calming effect on the brain, as well as being helpful for some hard-to-treat conditions including epilepsy and fibromyalgia. It's worth noting that CBD takes a while to integrate into the system, so give it a month or two of consistent use before deciding if it is helpful for you.

Melatonin is also a useful supplement, but is not commonly available in the UK (although you can find it from online pharmacies if you submit a request relating to sleep disturbance).

My Nightly Wind-Down Routine

A great day starts the night before, so I try to stick to this wind-down routine each and every night to wake up well:

As well as setting a morning alarm, I set an alarm to remind me it's time to start winding down for bed. This is usually 9pm, when I'll switch off my email and social media and limit my screen time. Late-night Netflix is an occasional treat, not an everyday habit. Instead, I'll read from the printed page or listen to an audio book or podcast. I drink herbal tea most evenings, something soporific

Bedded bliss

I recently discovered eucalyptus fibre sheets and duvet covers and have been impressed by how much of a difference these make to the quality of my sleep. Cool in the summer, cosy in the winter, my new-found bed friends are supremely comfortable as well as being easy-care. Beneath my bottom sheet, I also have a new addition. I first discovered 'grounding' when I spent time barefoot outdoors and felt better for it (see page 38). Over the years I have become more convinced by the (limited) science, so much so that I now sleep on a grounding sheet. There's not much hard science for sounder sleep, reduced cellular inflammation and reduced oxidative stress, but clinical evidence isn't always the acid test when it comes to whether or not something works. In my own experience, sleeping on top of a grounding sheet is a bio-hack that's hard to prove, but works anyway. I also like sleeping under a weighted blanket as the pressure promotes the production of serotonin, encouraging relaxation and sounder sleep.

such as valerian, chamomile or passionflower – or a combination of all three.

I take 120g magnesium glycinate half an hour or so before bed, either as a capsule or in a powdered warm, milky drink mix. If I'm going through an especially stressful time or my 'monkey brain' is jumping around, I'll also take L-theanine and vitamin B6, nick-named the 'chill pill' for its soothing, anti-anxiety properties. I'm also a fan of herbal sleeping tinctures (see Useful Resources, page 311). The amino acid glycine is also a useful addition to help sleep. And always – without fail – I sprinkle a few drops of neat lavender essential oil on my pillow (I travel with a bottle in my bag), shown to help sedate the brain. I don't bother with expensive sleep sprays, just a few drops of neat essential oil, which doesn't stain the pillow.

I'm also particular about the sartorial practicalities of sleep. I wear a soft bamboo fibre nightie or PJs that cover my shoulders so I don't get cold, but try to sleep with the window open and heating turned down, as we need cool temperatures to sleep better. I have blackout blinds *and* curtains to remove even the slightest chink of light that might keep me awake, and unplug any electric lights, or simply cover up any light sources (I travel with a roll of black tape to mask any annoying LED lights I can't easily unplug).

Last but not least, I sleep with a bite guard to reduce my stress-related molar grinding, which leads to temporomandibular joint (TMJ) issues, jaw pain, neck tension and headaches. Interestingly, TMJ is more common among midlife women, linked to oestrogen decline during menopause. I've tried many types in the past, including expensive custom-made bite guards, but find the inexpensive DenTek Ready-Fit Disposable Dental Guards work the best. The pack says they're disposable, but I clean and reuse each one many times before replacing. A bite guard won't necessarily stop jaw clenching, but it does help reduce its severity (and protect the teeth). More recently, I've also started mouth taping – sticking a small piece of skin-friendly tape over my lips to keep them together while I sleep. This simple trick means you can only breathe through your nose (shown to be more restful and even reduces snoring) . . .

Oh, and I leave my phone outside my bedroom door, so I'm not tempted by any late-night scrolling.

My bedside box of tricks

- Earplugs: the soft, silicone ones are comfiest for sleep. Mine are moulded to fit my ears – a good investment if your ears are very sensitive (most audiology clinics can custom-make ear plugs using a simple wax mould of your inner ear).

- Sleep drops: my favourites include various combinations of Montmorency cherry, L-theanine, inositol, Passiflora, valerian, scullcap, hops . . . all excellent for encouraging a deeper night's sleep.

- Facial oil: I prefer unscented oils on my face at night as I rely on lavender oil for a bedtime aroma. My bedside box houses an organic rosehip seed oil, good for rubbing into my jaw and neck to relax tense muscles as well as nourish dry skin overnight. I also rub some on the backs of my hands and into my nails to strengthen them.

- Notepad and pencil: last but not least, a notepad and pencil to get thoughts out of my brain and onto paper. Telling my brain that although problems exist, it doesn't need to dwell on them right now, which allows my mind to switch off.

Sleep is part of our round-the-clock wellness and needs to be actively scheduled and prepared for. Getting the environment right is important, as well as establishing a regular wind-down evening routine. Don't think that you can just flop into bed exhausted at the end of a busy day and flick the body's 'off' switch. A really good, deep, restful and restorative night's sleep requires a bit more thoughtful prep and care. It's worth it.

Healthy hacks

- Remember, how we start our day affects how well we sleep at night. Set your circadian rhythm up for success by getting some natural light on your skin and in your eyes as close to dawn as possible – every day.
- Magnesium is one of the most important supplements when it comes to better sleep. Take it 30 minutes before nodding off for best effect.
- Get a good bedtime routine going and stick to it: no screens two hours before bed (or wear blue light blocking glasses), use ear plugs and an eye shade if needed to block noise and light, sprinkle lavender oil on your pillow and keep the bedroom temperature cool.

CHAPTER 11

The Power of Connection

Strengthening our social ties and staying in touch and well connected with our circle of friends and family has a powerful effect on how we age. Many studies have shown that living in a community, be that physical or on a spiritual, faith-centred level, greatly increases our chances of living well for longer. Human beings are designed to be social creatures, not live in isolation and, as I mentioned in the opening pages, loneliness can literally be a killer. Social isolation significantly increases our risk of premature death from all causes, right up there with the more obvious risk factors of smoking, obesity and lack of exercise. A 2020 study by the National Academies of Sciences, Engineering, and Medicine associated loneliness with a 50 per cent increased risk of dementia, as well as rapidly rising rates of heart disease and stroke. Of course, some of us prefer our own company and are quite happy to live alone, but there is a big difference between being alone and being lonely. As we'll explore a bit later in this chapter, being happy in our own skin is important and we shouldn't need the company of others to complete us, but that feeling of being isolated is something else altogether.

When we talk about the important relationships in our lives, we tend to focus on the romantic kind involving husbands, other halves or life partners. But connections with our wider community are vitally important too. This can be our neighbours, work colleagues, faith community and fellow hobbyists as well as old friends. Chances are that at this stage of our lives, we don't feel much need to be going out to make new friends, so it's time to take stock of those who've been part of our inner circle for many years – those whom we truly value. Hopefully, we can all call to mind a few names of those we share private in-jokes with, those we could turn to in a crisis – or be there for them when they need a shoulder to cry or lean on. As we age, dramatic life changes are more likely to happen, such as divorce, health concerns, redundancy, debt or even the death of someone close to us. These significant events make it all the more important to nurture the protective friendship framework of those we've grown to love and trust. If this has made you think of a few special people in your life, whose friendship and wisdom you value, why not let them know right now? A simple phone call to say just that or, better yet, a handwritten card or letter to tell them how you feel and how much you appreciate them being in your life, however far away, is not only heart-warming to receive, you'll feel all the better for it too.

Getting Romance Right

I feel hesitant writing here on how to have a successful relationship, having been divorced twice. But, over my lifetime, I've had plenty of experience of how relationships work – and lived through dark times when they don't. I've learnt much from my connections with talented therapists and relationship counsellors I've worked with, both personally as well as professionally, and there are a few key points I'd like to pass on.

If you're lucky enough to be living in a loving relationship, it's important to acknowledge and treasure this. Growing old with someone you love and who loves you back is one of life's greatest gifts, but it rarely just 'happens'.

> **As with anything worth having,**
> **a successful relationship**
> **requires time, energy, thought,**
> **care and commitment.**

It's not exceptionally hard, but too many marriages break down when one or both partners don't put in the work. Sharing quality time is an easy win and, for those whose older children may have flown the nest, this can be the perfect time to sit down for a chat and a mutual think about how your lives may look from now on. If you're not already doing this, most relationship counsellors say a weekly date night with your significant other is foundational. Taking a moment in the week to focus on time shared between just the two of you presents the perfect opportunity to draw closer to each other and share mutual interests (or explore the other person's). Find the confidence to have conversations that redefine your romantic relationship, especially if sex has become an issue (more on this below). If that feels a bit awkward, start with open-ended questions such as 'How do you feel about our sex life?' or 'I miss our intimacy and would love to regain what we had – is that something you'd like too?' These open-ended questions can be a helpful starting-off point without being accusatory or threatening.

Having a much-loved life partner is both a blessing and a joy, but it may be that you're widowed, experienced heartbreak or been plunged into unexpected singledom. This hits hard at any age, but especially when you've been used to the company of another for many years, and it's important to acknowledge and honour this loss. Allow yourself the time to grieve, but do reach out for help and support from those around you and share how you feel. It won't take the pain away, but it will help diminish it to a level where you feel more able to cope. I've included some helpful resources for this at the back of the book (see page 308).

For those of you currently coming through a relationship breakdown or divorce, I sympathise. I've been there – and it's not an easy path to walk. However, a helpful thing psychotherapist Lucy Beresford taught me was to reframe how I thought about having had two 'failed marriages'. She picked me up on this when I mentioned my own experience and pointed out that as each one had lasted around 17 years, they could hardly be described as failures. I replied by saying that I hadn't got married only to get divorced later and that I took the vows, ''til death do us part' very seriously. She then, very gently, said that this did not have to mean the physical death of a person, it could also be applied to the death of a relationship. I found that profoundly helpful as yes, in both cases, my relationships had died, as we had grown and changed in ways not anticipated. But just because we had changed, this did not necessarily mean these relationships had been total failures. Both had enjoyed many positive life experiences and joyful moments,

The art of communication

I think it's fortunate for my fellow midlife women that we live in the times we do now when it comes to navigating the world of romance, marriage and loving partnerships. There's so much more open dialogue than when I was growing up and a vastly greater awareness of what is expected by our partners – and what we should expect in return. There's more acceptance and encouragement for open communication, without it becoming awkward or confrontational. And if I've learnt one thing in my love life, it is that communication is the cornerstone of it all.

The brilliant psychotherapist Lucy Beresford was so helpful here when we spoke on my podcast show and has a great take on how to make relationships work better. She says it's important for couples to have at least an annual review of how things are going, to talk without judgement about how they're feeling, what is going well, what they love and would like more of – and what is causing them unhappiness or concern. Just as we're comfortable with the idea of an end-of-term school report or an annual work review, so we should also set aside a specific time to talk to our partners to discuss how things are between us. This gives both parties the chance to voice small concerns or potential worries before they escalate. It's also a chance to celebrate the hurdles that have been overcome, the family challenges that have been met and dealt with together and to give thanks and praise where it's due.

I'm not entirely sure this helpful strategy would have 'saved' either of my own marriages, but it would have at least flagged up some fundamental concerns much earlier on and saved a good deal of heartache.

which should be remembered and honoured, not least because five extraordinary and wonderful children have been born into the world as a result. So, if you feel as though you've somehow 'failed' because things didn't turn out in the way you'd hoped or expected, do take heart.

We can't change what's happened to us, but we can change the way we feel about it.

Sex Talk

Now, I'm not a sex therapist, so am not qualified to talk at length about the ins and outs (excuse the pun) of a fulfilling and satisfying sex life. There are plenty of others who do this brilliantly – sexwise.org.uk, askwithoutshame.org, quantumsex.co.uk, and the (very) explicit Sex with Emily podcast and website spring to mind. However, there is a clear connection between sex, wellbeing and ageing well. A happy, relaxed and satisfying sex life is surely a joyful relationship goal, but often one that's hard to sustain over time. The pressures of work, children, illness and more can push sex down the priority list, despite most relationship counsellors highlighting its importance. Of course, sex is not essential and there are many couples who have a very happy life together without even sleeping in the same bedroom. As long as this is an entirely mutual agreement then fair enough. But if we're able to maintain and enjoy a physical relationship over many years, warm up a cold one or even start a new one in later life, this brings with it so many wellness benefits.

On a purely physical level, sex has plenty of healthspan strong points. When we connect skin-on-skin, our blood pressure lowers and our hormones are encouraged into better balance. For women, penetrative sex strengthens their pelvic floor, improves bladder control and helps prevent prolapse, as orgasm causes contractions in the pelvic-floor muscles (the more often we can do this, the better). It also strengthens our abdominal muscles (counting as exercise!) and even improves our immune systems, as studies show that those who have regular sex take fewer sick days due to greater protective antibody activity. Those having sex once a week or more have been shown to have more immunoglobulin A (IgA) in their saliva, which is the first line of antibody defence against many illnesses, including human papillomavirus, or HPV. Women who remain sexually active after the menopause are also less likely to have significant vaginal atrophy (where the tissue lining of the vagina becomes drier, more fragile and prone to splitting) – a good case for use it or lose it. Orgasm can also block pain as it releases a hormone that helps raise our pain thresholds. There's a physical reason why we sleep better after having sex too, as orgasm releases the hormone prolactin, making us feel more relaxed, safer and sleepier. Sexual intimacy also reduces anxiety and depression, improving our overall state of mind. Achieving orgasm (whether with someone else or solo) activates potent neurotransmitters in the brain, principally oxytocin, nicknamed the love hormone, and having sex (especially orgasm, but even without) floods the brain with oxytocin, filling our entire bodies with a warm, rosy glow. Masturbation does the same, albeit to a lesser degree than sex within a loving relationship. Sex doesn't have to be all about penetration to feel these benefits either. Positive and powerful neurotransmitters are released when we kiss, feel our skin being stroked or a hand being held, or when we engage in intimate talking.

However, for many midlife women especially, there may be many barriers to entry (sorry!) when it comes to having sex, ranging from the physical to emotional and mental-health demons. If you're struggling, it's worth talking to a relationship counsellor or taking a look at some of the free online resources I've included on page 308. So many studies show that the more sex we have, the better our bodies respond. For those who haven't had sex in a while though, the thought of that first foray back into the bedroom can be a bit overwhelming. Lack of sex due to pain, disappointment, violence or other forms of trauma are all reasons why we can become avoidant, and are signs we should reach out for help and guidance.

For many midlife women, declining hormones can definitely reduce desire. As testosterone levels fall, so does libido. We may simply feel less inclined, which is why testosterone replacement is recommended as a simple, safe and effective therapy. Along with the upsides for sexual activity, the attendant reported benefits include a lifting of mood, clearing of brain fog, improved memory (especially word recall) and greater overall muscle tone – all positive things that are likely to make us more generally 'in the mood'.

Once we actually feel like having sex, it's important to make it comfortable and easy. Replacement oestrogen helps with vaginal dryness, restoring the natural pH balance within the vagina and helping to prevent vaginal atrophy (alongside reducing UTIs and urinary incontinence). For those not on HRT, something as simple as a localised vaginal oestrogen cream or pessary can make all the difference and is considered very safe, as the oestrogen stays within the vagina and does not spread around the body. For those taking HRT, adding in a bit of localised vaginal oestrogen may also be helpful for improving vaginal health when used alongside oestrogen gels, sprays, patches or pills, and can be prescribed on top of HRT. It's amazing the difference this can make to your comfort. Oh, and don't forget to use a lubricant too – liberal lube is a midlife sex secret worth sharing. Choose a formula with a pH that matches the vagina (it will say so on the pack) to moisturise and lubricate intimate tissues, but watch out for ingredients that can cause irritation and trigger UTIs, notably propylene glycol and glycerine, a sugar that will feed vaginal thrush. A sex therapist recently shared with me the art of 'slide and glide' where each partner uses a different formulation, one oil-based, the other water-based (each can be applied to either partner) to increase the degree and duration of the experience.

Toxic Truths

There are many reasons why relationships break down and come to an end. These days, we're hopefully more aware of how another's behaviour might be affecting us. Phrases such as gaslighting, coercive control, emotional abuse, toxic masculinity and narcissism have become more widely recognised.

A partner's negative behaviour leaves its mark, especially when repeated over time. Be vigilant for the early warning signs of being undermined, those red flags that damage, such as constant criticism, the flashes of unprovoked anger and lack of support that can build and ultimately boil over. However, the signs of these can be cunning and may build subtly over time, like a frog being boiled in water so slowly it doesn't realise the danger, and there's a real chance we may not even realise what is happening.

So how do we recognise a toxic relationship, let alone deal with it? Sometimes it takes a friend or family member to make us aware of what is going on. It can be helpful to turn to someone close to you who can see your situation with objective clarity; someone trusted who is able to stand back and discern the toxic patterns of behaviour you might otherwise be oblivious to when you're in the thick of it. If you suspect this is happening in your relationship, ask a close friend for their honest opinion. And if you see it happening to someone you care about, don't be afraid to gently speak up, even if it seems a hard subject to broach. In my experience, the handful of good friends I have raised this with as a possibility have all been appreciative – if not immediately, then most definitely in the longer term. A good friend is someone who has your back, even if that means engaging in a potentially difficult conversation about a relationship.

Should I Stay or Should I Go?

This is a question that often gets raised during midlife. It may be that you've grown apart, the family dynamic has shifted as children leave home or personal situations have changed. Perhaps you've been betrayed by your partner – or maybe you've been the betrayer. Can these situations ever be worked through and resolved? From talking to relationship counsellors on this, the answer is yes, but it does take effort and commitment – on both sides.

Co-dependency is common in long-term relationships but is unhealthy when it allows self-destructive behaviour and poor mental health, or if it holds you back from reaching your true potential. Of course, we're designed to be social beings, ideally with a supportive and loving spouse or partner, but this is not always either possible or something we want.

Ultimately, the answer to the stay-or-go question is complex and individual, but my view is that it needs to be considered in light of how you feel about yourself as much as how you feel about your 'other half', which brings me on to the importance of finding your purpose.

Finding Your Purpose

Sometimes we stay with our significant others because we're scared of being alone, so the first step to being happy and finding a fulfilling relationship is to feel happy and fulfilled in our own skin. After my relatively recent divorce, I spent several years living on my own, getting to better know myself and discover what makes me, Liz the singleton, tick. I learnt to enjoy doing things solo, activities that I would never have otherwise considered. I went to the theatre on my own, booking a pre-performance supper for one and enjoying an interval drink without any other company but my own. While scary at first, I realised that I actually enjoyed my evening out. I didn't need anyone else to sit beside me to have a great evening. If you've never had a date with yourself, give it a try, even if you're in a relationship – you may be surprised by how much you enjoy it.

During my own 'wilderness' years, I came to realise how important it is to love yourself before being loved by others.

You shouldn't need anyone
else to complete you.

It is truly wonderful if and when you find someone who adds to your sense of completeness, but it needn't be a condition of your own happiness.

So far, this book has been about internally bio-hacking our way into a better second half of life. But ultimately, there has to be a reason that we do this. Why do we get out of bed in the morning? Why are you and I here? Is it to survive or thrive? Do we exist simply to be or are we here to leave something of benefit behind, to validate why we were given space on this precious planet? I believe the answer to these profoundly deep and meaningful questions lies in finding our purpose.

Purpose goes a long way in helping make sense of it all. As I said at the outset, by the time we reach midlife and beyond it's very easy to have lost ourselves, unaware of the values that truly define us. One advantage of growing older is to have a little more time away from the pressures of work and family to consider this – and act before the chance passes us by. No one wants to end their life thinking, Was that it?

Now's the time to dig deep into what has got us to where we are in life, what has shaped who we really are, what drives, motivates and ultimately, fulfils us. Do we merely want a good life – or a meaningful one?

Gratitude goals
Let's begin with a look at gratitude, a trait that goes a long way in framing how we feel about life. We all have something to be grateful for, no matter what stones have been thrown at us

– from the air in our lungs to fresh water coming out of a tap, to a safe bed to sleep in, family, friendships and so much more besides. If you don't already keep a gratitude journal, I highly recommend starting one now. It doesn't have to be a daily record, it could be something as simple as making a note at the end of each week of some good things you've experienced and are truly grateful for.

Taking a moment to write down a few of the things we're thankful for is a powerful mental health habit worth having.

It's easy to lose sight of gratitude, to be dangerously discontent, feeding anger and bitterness. Maybe life hasn't turned out as we'd hoped or planned, but it's important not to lose perspective of what we *do* have. The modern world is masterful at breeding resentment and envy. We're constantly told that what we have is not enough, that we need to be better than we are, more success-ful, own the latest life-enhancing gadget, model of car, brand of handbag . . . We're led to believe that these things somehow define who we are or how we feel. Stepping off that treadmill, escaping the matrix and appreciating what we actually have (the really important stuff) frees our hearts and minds for what actu-ally really matters.

If you're in a loving, long-term relationship right now, recognise your good fortune. Don't take your other half for granted, and if you really do love them, don't forget to tell them so! Reinstating the romantic gestures of your courting days goes a long way to showing the other person how much you care and are grateful for their companionship. Slip a cheeky note into their lunchbox or sports bag to make them smile, or perhaps send a simple text message saying 'thinking of you and hope your day is going well' to show you're thinking about them and care about their wellbeing. If your significant other does something special for you, be sure to acknowledge this. Saying 'I had a great time; I so appreciate what you did', is much more likely to make it a repeat occurrence. Genuine gratitude makes us feel valued and acknowledged, so don't hold back the praise. We're never too old for a bit of affirmation and affection-fuelled consideration.

Gratitude is also a superpower that improves longevity and supports the immune system. Studies show that feeling thankful improves quality of sleep, boosts our moods, decreases our risk of depression and anxiety and can even help ease physical pain and risk of disease.

Make a contribution

The knowledge that we can and do make a difference to the lives of others is one of the best ways to live more happily. Becoming a contributor and developing a sense of belonging is what makes a long-lived life worth living. They say it is greater to give than to receive and I have personally found this to be true. That warm, fuzzy feeling you get when you lend a hand to those in need or support someone with a hug, kind words or physical assistance produces powerfully uplifting endorphins in the brain.

There are many life stages and those of us lucky enough to reach older age are the fortunate ones. Our first stage of life is spent growing into our skin and then potentially growing careers, relationships and often children. Between our thirties and fifties we're developing and expanding who we are. Later life is the time to discover the beauty of giving back, to reap the benefits of all we have learnt, to pass on knowledge, to utilise our wisdom and skills. In return, we can achieve genuine fulfilment and ultimate contentment, especially if we allow ourselves to follow our true passions.

When looking back at my life so far, I am especially struck by the work of palliative-care nurse Bronnie Ware, who spent many years looking after those who are dying. She captured some of these deathbed insights in a brilliant book called *The Top Five Regrets of the Dying*, which I highly recommend. You can't fail but be moved by these profoundly raw and honest conversations. They certainly made me pause and reflect on my own work and life's purpose – as well as my relationships, both past and present. I suspect they'll do the same for you too, so I'll share some of the wisdom here. According to Bronnie, the most common regret was 'I wish I'd lived a life true to myself and not what other people expected of me'. The second was 'I wish I hadn't worked so hard', followed by 'I wish I'd had the courage to express my feelings', 'I wish I'd stayed in touch with my friends' and, finally (and perhaps most heartbreakingly), 'I wish I'd allowed myself to be happier'. Allow those words of regret to sink in, and I defy anyone not to be stirred to make shifts in life for the better, while there's still time. The truths people share on their deathbed powerfully teach us about how we should be living our lives now.

Play to your strengths

So how best to live more authentically, with greater meaning and purpose? We all have strengths that lead us to develop these opportunities. I admire the work of the bestselling psychologist Dr

A BETTER SECOND HALF

Martin Seligman, who describes 24 personal strengths to help discover meaning and purpose. You'll find his free online survey at viacharacter.org where you can take the free VIA Strengths Survey, a 25-minute exercise that ranks your strengths – character traits such as originality, courage, honesty, kindness, justice, leadership, mercy, humour, integrity and more – from top to bottom. The ranking reflects how you rate your strengths and how much of each you possess. Your top five results are the ones to pay attention to and help find ways to build a more purpose-filled future.

In his book *Authentic Happiness* Dr Seligman writes 'Identify your signature strengths and choose work that lets you use them every day. Recraft your work to use your signature strengths more. Release your own potential for flow.' The results of others I know taking this test reveal strengths of courage, patience, empathy and more. In some cases, this has encouraged them to volunteer as helpers in the prison service, children's reading assistants and, for one housebound friend, training as a phone counsellor for the Samaritans. Volunteering is a wonderful way to build social connections and add purpose and meaning to life – and we all have something to give, be it time, money or talent.

Empathy is a great relationship builder and goes a long way in reconnecting with those we may have unwittingly grown apart from.

Having spent some quality time alone with myself, I'm more aware than ever of my personal values, how I like to spend my time and what really interests me. I've also grown to appreciate my friendships and have given more of my time to friends, my parents and my children as a result. If I am in a close relationship with someone now, it is because I choose to be, not because I feel there is something missing or a gap that needs filling for me to be whole.

If you're in a loving relationship, treasure it and keep it safe. Guard it as you would your most valuable possessions. Ultimately, though, be discerning about who and what you give your time to. Recognising unacceptable patterns of behaviour within relation-ships (of all kinds) is vitally important for your overall health and happiness. Just because you've hit midlife or beyond doesn't mean that this must be your lot. A bad relationship or marriage is not something you simply have to learn to live with. That may be how you're feeling now, but you deserve better, and having a better second half is all about recognising the opportunity for change and acting on it. Relish the prospect and the possibilities – that's what this book is all about.

Healthy hacks
- Take stock of your relationship by suggesting a review with your significant other. How is it working for you? What posi-tive changes would you like to make? Speak these out or, if that's too scary, write them down and share in a letter.
- Sex-wise, consider ways to improve your vaginal health, such as pelvic floor exercises to strengthen your vagina which will improve sexual satisfaction as well as having other pelvic-health benefits.

- Strengthen ties with your communities, at work, in your neighbourhood and with your friendship group. Recognise friends or partners who radiate or drain, call out the crazy-makers and give those you truly love and value a bit more of your time.

CHAPTER 12

Beauty Bio-Hacks

Beauty bio-hacking can be a real game changer when it comes to living longer and looking well, with many quick and simple wins. In this chapter, I've included a few things I've grown to love to look well for longer.

Pro-Ageing Supplements

I've already mentioned some of the amazing pro-ageing supplements that help increase healthspan as well as lifespan, including glutathione, CoQ10 and spermidine (all of which I take daily – see pages 64, 66 and 183). But there are a few others worthy of a mention here.

Resveratrol

Outlined in my chat about the benefits of red wine on page 204, this potent plant polyphenol is mostly found in dark chocolate, red and purple berries as well as red grape skins, and is one of my must-haves. Resveratrol is a highly potent antioxidant, reducing cell damage as we age, activating those sirtuins that protect our DNA (see page 53). Resveratrol protects ageing brains against diseases such as Alzheimer's, guards against cancer and lowers blood pressure. Supplementing with resveratrol when combined with a high-fat diet has been shown to improve cholesterol balance and help with weight loss. It also helps with insulin sensitivity as well as improving our response to glucose.

NAD+

NAD+ is one of the more recently discovered bio-hacks when it comes to longevity – and the science is solid. NAD+ is a co-enzyme found in all living cells. Its job is to assist over 500 enzymatic reactions. We create NAD+ within our cells from niacin and other vitamin B3 derivatives found in foods, such as beef, eggs, avocado, salmon and dark leafy greens, when combined with enzymes and other nutrients, such as alpha-lipoic acid and NMN. Because it's created within our cells, it's not possible to effectively supplement directly with NAD+, but we can give the body the ingredients it needs to build its own supplies. Supplementing with the nutrients that support NAD+ production (notably NMN, alpha-lipoic acid and quercetin), increases the body's own production. Exercise can also give our levels a boost, with two sessions of resistance training each week for ten weeks significantly increasing NAD+ levels in untrained adults. Autophagy, or intense fasting, also triggers the production of NAD+ (see page 57). If you take NAD+-supporting supplements you can expect to feel more awake, have more energy and feel less hungry. Those taking regular NAD+ boosters also report smoother, younger-looking skin as a result – I include myself here.

NAD+ boosters are one of the most
powerful resources we have for
improving our longevity and supporting
better health and beauty as we age.

Quercetin

From the Latin word *Quercetum*, meaning oak forest, quercetin is
another antioxidant flavonoid found in red-skinned fruits and
vegetables. I gave it a brief mention earlier as a helpful remedy for
hay fever as it helps regulate our histamine response, but it has
powerful pro-ageing, beauty benefits too as it dampens down
inflammation. I now take quercetin year-round as it regulates the
SIRT1 gene, linked with longevity. There's a strong case for quercetin helping to ward off many of the degenerative diseases associated with ageing, including Alzheimer's, Parkinson's, Huntington's,
depression, osteoporosis, hardening of the arteries and CHD.
Quercetin also has powerful antiviral properties and was one of
the nutrients highlighted as being helpful for the treatment and
prevention of Covid-19.

Making Sense of Methylation

Many important nutrients influence how well cells age, but
these are all dependent on how our genes are expressed.
Genetics influences longevity, but we can help activate how our
genes express themselves (the process of epigenetics that
changes how the body 'reads' our DNA). DNA methylation is an
important epigenetic process our cells use to control how genes
express themselves.

Put simply, methylation acts as the conductor of our biological orchestra, controlling the expression of our genes. When methylation is working optimally, it turns unnecessary genes off and ensures vital genes are on, playing their part in maintaining our wellbeing. Importantly, methylation helps eliminate toxins, produce energy and synthesise neurotransmitters, which orchestrate mood, focus, sleep and stress response. Think of it as a cleaning ritual for your cellular wellbeing, not unlike a deep, cleansing facial for your skin clearing away debris and giving you a glow. Just as the skin can show signs of imbalance though, so too can the methylation processes. Lifestyle factors such as stress, poor diet, lack of exercise and environmental toxins all disrupt this cellular harmony.

Maintaining methylation balance is integral to overall wellbeing, but, as with most things, gets harder for our bodies as we age. Regular exercise, a balanced diet rich in methylation-supporting nutrients such as B vitamins, folate and amino acids, plus getting better sleep, all help ensure our bodies' methylation processes are finely tuned and harmonious. When we lack these, the body becomes de-methylated, which impacts how our genes function – and needs to be avoided! Methylation is the ultimate wellness practice for our genes, so make a note of this important word as we'll be hearing more about it in the future.

How Collagen Supports the Skin

As well as nutrients to support gene expression and make the most of my methylation, I also take collagen for my ageing skin and connective tissues. From the age of 25 our collagen levels start to fall and this loss shows up as fine lines, skin wrinkling and stiffer joints. Collagen is the main structural protein in the body, especially for the skin, as well as the main component of joint cartilage (supplementing can help with arthritic joints too). Collagen is also found in our bones, helping tensile strength, stimulating the production of new bone cells and improving bone density (especially important for midlife women and beyond), as well as being an important part of cardiac tissue and gut lining.

There are several different types on the market, including drinks, capsules and powders. The best ones contain collagen peptides or hydrolysed collagen of a low 'dalton' weight, ideally below 2 kDa, to be better absorbed. However, collagen liquids and powders are broken down in the stomach into their component amino acids, so their peptides are unlikely to get absorbed intact. That's not to say they don't have an effect as their amino acids are useful building blocks for the body to make its own supplies by rejoining the amino acids, but our ability to do this reduces with age, so these are not the most reliable way of taking collagen, especially when we're older. I prefer collagen supplements contained within a capsule clinically proven to withstand the intense acidity of the stomach. Their contents are more likely to reach the small intestine intact, where the pH changes, the capsule dissolves and the peptides are then released. Because some collagen capsules reach the small intestine intact, fewer peptides are needed to have an effect, which is why you need much less than larger scoops of the powdered or liquid form to see an effect.

All collagen comes from animal sources as collagen does not exist in the plant kingdom. They tend to be either made from bovine (beef) sources or marine (usually fish skin). There's no such thing as vegan collagen, although some brands make vegan supplements that support the body's own ability to make collagen. These may include vitamins E and C as well as hyaluronic acid and zinc.

When you start taking collagen, allow around a month before seeing the difference in your skin, followed by stronger nails and less painful joints. Collagen supplements help improve hair strength too, although this takes longer because hair has to grow. See Useful Resources, page 312 for the brand I buy.

Pro-ageing Skincare

As co-founder of one of the most successful British beauty brands of all time, I'm always asked about my own skincare routine. Despite no longer having any connection with my eponymous brand, I still use its original cream cleanser and muslin cloth night and morning – and have found nothing to beat it. The very first product I ever created (I still have the notepad with my original formulae jottings), I'm proud that Cleanse & Polish has stood the test of time. Over the years, I've added other products into my daily routine for their specific pro-ageing benefits. Part of my job is to review skincare innovations, so I'm always trialling something new on my skin, but these are the key ingredients I come back to time and again:

Azelaic acid

Used to treat acne and rosacea, I've added azelaic acid into my nightly skincare routine as it can reduce pigmentation. It contains a natural tyrosine inhibitor, which helps control melanin production in skin cells and I've found it effective for reducing age spots on my face and the backs of my hands. Many skin creams contain azelaic acid and it's well tolerated by sensitive skins.

Hyaluronic acid

Found naturally in the skin, hyaluronic acid can hold up to 1,000 times its weight in water, keeping joints and connective tissues plump and smooth. It declines with age, so taking supplements is useful for our faces as well as our mobility. Increasingly found in skincare, several different molecular weights are used in moisturisers, designed to penetrate to varying levels. Hyaluronic acid is also available as an injectable (see page 298) and is one of the main skincare ingredients (both internal and external) I advise for those with drier, more mature skin.

Niacinamide

Also known as nicotinamide, this type of vitamin B3 is helpful for inflammatory skin conditions, including acne and eczema, evening skin tone and helping prevent blotchiness. In skincare, this nutrient helps build keratin proteins in the skin, strengthening the epidermis to prevent moisture loss. Niacinamide also helps the skin's lipidic ceramide barrier, especially useful for more mature skin as poor barrier function is one reason skin becomes drier with age. It helps repair sun damage and 5 per cent concentrations have been shown to reduce age spots too. It's most often found in serums and night creams, and is another key ingredient I like to see in a formula.

Retinol

These compounds are derived from vitamin A and are highly effective at plumping, smoothing and brightening the skin. Each type works by reducing the breakdown of collagen and speeding up skin cell turnover, so fresh young skin cells are encouraged nearer the skin's surface, reducing fine lines and wrinkles. Tretinoin is the best known retinol, used since the sixties in acne treatments, but only available on prescription. Many aesthetic doctors and dermatologists use retinols as a pro-ageing treatment, but you'll find lower-strength versions in high street skincare too. The form of retinol in over-the-counter face creams needs to be converted by the body into retinoic acid (the stronger stuff prescribed by doctors), so it takes longer to see its effects, but the difference to the skin can be dramatic. Retinols can make the skin more sensitive to sunlight (although the newer formulations are photostable), so are best used at night and followed by a moisturiser and sunscreen in the morning. You don't need much – a pea-sized amount is sufficient for the whole face and you can also mix with a moisturiser to weaken their skin-flaking effect if your skin is very sensitive. Useful for the neck and upper chest area too.

Rosehip oil

I've a long-standing love of this natural plant oil, mainly due to its high vitamin E content, but also because it contains natural carotenoids (antioxidants that help guard against cell damage) and trans retinoic acid, a retinoid that helps renew skin cells. Not as powerful as retinol itself, rosehip oil still makes an excellent facial oil and is the one I use neat on my own skin for facial massage (especially for gua sha, see page 301). It's especially soothing for sensitive skin and can help calm breakouts and minor skin irritations. Used regularly, rosehip oil helps fade scars and reduce skin discoloration. It's a lovely botanical plant oil; try adding a few drops of lavender, chamomile or neroli essential oil to make a fragrant body oil.

Tweakments

As well as skincare, I'm often asked about tweakments (non-surgical cosmetic treatments). There are so many new and interesting ways to 'tweak' the way our faces age, and during my 40 or so years in the beauty business I've tried a few – nothing drastic, but some have been beneficial.

LED-light and laser facials

LED-light and laser facials are non-invasive ways to stimulate collagen and tighten slackening skin, and are my go-tos these days. I'll have a laser facial treatment every three to four months and I use the Cellreturn Platinum LED face mask most nights before bed. Originally launched by my eldest daughter Lily, I think they make the best-in-class when it comes to LED light for beauty treatments, including hair loss. With a credible medical licence to prove its efficacy, this LED face mask works by using a specific frequency and strength of light that penetrates through the skin to stimulate collagen and elastin fibres beneath the epidermis. It really does work and I use it before bed as the red light frequency also encourages better sleep (blue light wakes us up, which is why using screens – phones, laptops, TV screens and so on – before bed is a bad idea). Cellreturn UK also has a 360-degree 'Neckle Ray Plus' which I also wear most days for 20 minutes or so to target my chin and neck. This is especially good as you simply slip it around your neck and go about your day unimpeded. Some days I'll use it twice . . . There are many LED mask brands on the market, and the most effective ones are those that are medical-grade and are inevitably pricey, but independent testing has shown

Cellreturn to come out top. I do genuinely consider this to be a worthwhile piece of pro-ageing kit and a valid investment.

Injectables

When it comes to injectables, the most well known are Botox and fillers, and I've experimented with both. Botox is a prescription only product so you should take medical advice before you have a botox procedure and make sure you only have it done by a licensed health professional. I don't use Botox very often and never in large amounts as I don't like having my facial expression frozen, but I do have a bit of 'baby Botox' (tiny amounts) in my forehead – not enough to 'freeze' it or to prevent me from wrinkling my brow, just enough to prevent deep furrows and wrinkles from forming. I don't want to look different or even much younger; I just want to look the same.

> The cost of Botox often depends on the amount used, so 'baby Botox' is a cheaper option and gives a more natural effect.

I have a higher dose of Botox injected into the masseter muscle of my right jaw twice a year to relax ingrained tension and reduce my night-time jaw clenching, which used to give me headaches (as well as impacting my teeth). Botox is a safe and highly effective way to immobilise muscles, preventing them from contracting, which is why it's such a good treatment for migraine and deeply held muscle tension too.

When it comes to fillers, these are excellent for areas of the face that have lost plumpness as collagen and elastin supplies decline. My own face is naturally quite plump and I find I can maintain this with collagen supplements, a high-fat and -protein diet and LED light, but if you've lost volume in your cheeks or lips, fillers can be a safe and effective way of replacing this.

More recently, I've been trialling a newer form of hyaluronic acid injections, where small amounts of this naturally occurring gooey substance are injected just beneath the skin to stimulate the body into producing more collagen. I've also tried needling with exosomes, the communication components of cells that are similar in activity to stem cells. Originally used by the medical profession for injecting into areas of the body in need of regeneration, such as an arthritic knee or injury-related site of pain, exosomes trigger the body's own production of fresh, young skin cells within the skin – helping the skin renew itself and encourage a more youthful cell structure. These can be microneedled into the skin (via tiny perforations) or injected just beneath the surface. Again, safe and effective, I like the way these work with the body's natural regeneration processes, instead of simply relying on an artificial filler. I've found both hyaluronic acid and exosomes to be especially good around the eye area for de-puffing and softening fine lines.

I believe the decision on whether or not to use injectables is entirely personal – your face, your choice. And if the results make you feel happier and more at ease with the visible signs of ageing when you look in the mirror, then why on earth not? I don't think we should be guilt-tripped if we decide to use them, or feel pressured to go down that path if we don't. Being in the public eye certainly increases the pressure of being judged by appearance, but I have many friends who simply want to look fresher, not as tired and 'less cross' by having a tweak or two. Fair enough I say.

Non-Surgical Face Lifters

As well as, or instead of, tweakments, there are many other non-invasive beauty hacks we can do at home. These are the ones I've found work best:

Dermablading

This uses a specific facial blade to literally shave away the fine baby hair on the face known as vellus. It's popular with Hollywood's A-listers before a red carpet event, and while I was sceptical at first, I am now hooked. You just need a disposable dermaplane (inexpensive and easily found online) to glide over freshly cleansed, lightly oiled skin (use your favourite facial oil or moisturiser) to whisk off the peachy fuzz along with dead epidermal skin cells. Especially good for midlife women whose faces can grow furrier with age, this simple, safe technique works really well (a good hack for eyebrow shaping too). And no, vellus hair doesn't grow back thicker or darker, it regrows in the same soft way as before. Tip: use a magnifying mirror, go slowly and gently, avoid any skin irritations and don't use any potentially irritating skincare afterwards, such as fruit acids or retinols. Follow with your usual serum and/or moisturiser.

Fasting

This may come as a surprise, but fasting can dramatically change the way your face looks – and not just by weight loss. When we fast for an extended period (72 hours or more), we trigger autophagy – as we've seen, a key player in optimising healthspan. Autophagy doubles as a beauty treatment by encouraging the body to 'eat' up cell debris and unwanted cellular debris, including dead skin cells and scar tissue. According to fasting pioneer Megan Ramos (who works alongside the godfather of intermittent fasting, Dr Jason Fung), she's seen surgical scarring magically melt away after periods of fasting, as the body literally digests unwanted tissue. I saw this for myself after a five-day fast at the Buchinger Wilhelmi clinic in Germany, when I was struck by how much my face had firmed up, so much so I was asked if I'd had a facelift (I haven't). Even shorter periods of intermittent fasting, such as the 16:8 protocol, reduces inflammation and puffiness, brightens the complexion and gives skin a more youthful glow. Yet another reason to give it a go.

Gua sha

I was taught this simple facial massage technique by the master practitioner Katie Brindle, who has excellent (free) online tutorials. It uses a smooth, flat, pebble-shaped tool made of quartz that you stroke in firm, precise movements over lightly oiled skin. Gua sha massage reduces puffiness by improving lymphatic drainage and brightens skin by boosting blood flow. It's brilliant first thing in the morning to 'wake up' the face and help with under-eye bags and jawline puffiness. You can also use gua sha on other areas of the body, especially for relieving muscle tension (I use it on my neck if I feel a headache coming on) and some acupuncturists and other TCM practitioners use it to help treat chronic pain and inflammation.

> **Beauty is more than what we put onto our skins; it starts from within as this is where we make our skin cells.**

Getting up earlier, looking at the early-morning sun, staying well hydrated, eating real food cooked from scratch, adding in a few key nutrients, TRE, taking exercise, having cold showers and meditation all give us a glow. No amount of skincare or beauty treatments can make up for poor health habits, but we can support our health and longevity with some simple, well-recognised beauty hacks to help us on the way to looking well for longer.

Beauty hacks
- Put the power of fasting into practice, not just TRE but the occasional 24-hour fast for tighter, brighter skin. Probably not enough to trigger autophagy, but helpful for reducing puffiness in the face.
- Add in a few internal skin-savers. The most potent of these for pro-ageing are collagen as well as resveratrol, quercetin and NAD+ boosters, the powerful anti-inflammatory antioxidants that protect ageing cells, so they behave in a more youthful way.
- Upgrade your skincare armoury with some of the newer ingredients proven to be powerfully pro-ageing, including retinols, azelaic acid and niacinamide. Use rosehip oil for gua sha or facial massage.

Final Note

As you step into your better second half, I hope I have managed to capture some of the principles I consider to be the most important as we age. It's no secret that, as we age, we value life more. We're more aware of our own mortality, especially as we lose people close to us and maybe have our own health battles to fight too. We observe the sharp reality that life in this world is short, and start to question what we have made of it so far and what the next half might look like. It really doesn't matter if we feel that opportunities have passed us by, though – this is no time for looking back at what might have been. Instead, it's the time to stretch forward to what is yet to come, to reach our full potential by being strong enough to achieve what it is that we really want in our remaining years. Can the next stage truly be filled with joy, energy, peace and productivity (even if the first half might not have been?). I really believe it can. For us all.

What patterns of behaviour have formed over the years that might need to change? Given your new-found energy, vitality and positivity from putting at least some of the takeaways in this book into practice, what opportunities now lie ahead?

Whatever age you are or whatever life stage you're at, right now is the only reality. We can't control the past. We can't predict the future. These do not define us. What's real is the here and now – and we alone have the power to choose how we respond to this actual moment in time.

I'll end by saying that I have learnt to accept the past and be optimistic about the future. But what matters, above all, is living well in this moment, right now.

Go well.

Liz ♥

Useful Resources

Liz Earle Wellbeing

The home of Liz Earle and her wellness team can be found at: lizearlewellbeing.com. Here you can also sign up to the *free* weekly newsletters. The *Liz Earle Wellbeing Show* podcast is available as a free download from all major podcast platforms, or the website.

- lizearlewellbeing
- @LizEarleWb
- @lizearlewellbeing
- @lizearlewellbeing

At-home health screening

BetterYou: betteryou.com
GlycanAge: glycanage.com
WomenWise: womenwise.health
Optimally Me: optimallyme.com

Alcohol support

Alcoholchange.org.uk
Alcoholics-anonymous.org.uk

Beauty
Cellreturn UK: cellreturn.co.uk
Highly effective LED face, hair and neck masks.

Hayo'u Method: hayoumethod.com
For gua sha tutorials and how-tos.

The Tweakments Guide: thetweakmentsguide.com
For advice on 'tweakments' and cosmetic surgery.

Brain health
Drug Science: drugscience.org.uk
For the latest research and the use of psychedelics, medical cannabis and more.

Cold-water swimming
The Outdoor Swimming Society: outdoorswimmingsociety.com
For details on where to find a cold-water group near you.

Exercise
NHS Couch to 5k app: nhs.uk/live-well/exercise/running-and-aerobic-exercises/get-running-with-couch-to-5k

Fasting
Buchinger Wilhelmi: buchinger-wilhelmi.com
Buchingher Wilhelmi clinics in both Germany and southern Spain are considered the best in the world for supervised fasting. They also have an excellent YouTube channel with tutorials and offer a comprehensive at-home DIY fasting box.

Functional medicine practitioners

Functional Medicine Associates: functional-medicine.associates
One of the UK's first and leading groups of functional medicine practitioners.

Nature Doc: naturedoc.com
Specialists in family and children's functional health, gut and mould issues.

Hooke: hooke.london
State of the art diagnostic testing, highest quality health screening, mind/body analysis and support.

The Institute for Functional Medicine: ifm.org
The world's largest referral network of accredited practitioners.

The Key Clinic: thekeyclinic.co.uk
Specialists in neurodiverse issues.

Genetic testing

Lifecode Gx: lifecodegx.com
Professional genotype analysis.

OptimallyMe: optimallyme.com
Tests include epigenetic clock (biological versus chronological age) and NAD+ analysis.

Meditation

London Meditation Centre: londonmeditationcentre.com
For Vedic meditation workshops and tuition.

Menopause matters
Balance app: balance-menopause.com/balance-app
This free menopause app is available globally for all women to track their hormones and access evidence-based information relating to peri-menopause, menopause and post-menopause. I highly recommend it.

Newson Health: newsonhealth.co.uk
The leading independent menopause support clinics in the UK for in-person or online appointments, Newson Health offers a wide range of treatments from HRT to holistic therapies. Consultations with special-ist input are also available for those who have had breast cancer. This is also the place to go if you're considering replacement testosterone for low libido, alongside discussions with your GP. They also run a not-for profit research centre and have an excellent educational course for clinicians (and anyone else interested) at: newson-health.teachable.com

The Menopause Charity: themenopausecharity.org
On a mission to deliver trusted information and education.

Relationships
For relationship counselling, see:
Lucy Beresford: lucyberesford.com
James Earl: jamesearl.com

For grief support, see:
Cruse Bereavement Support: cruse.org.uk

For advice on sex, see:
Ask Without Shame: askwithoutshame.org
David Brown: quantumsex.co.uk
Sexwise: sexwise.org.uk
Sex with Emily: sexwithemily.com

Further Reading

- *A Statin-Free Life: A Revolutionary Life Plan for Tackling Heart Disease – Without the Use of Statins* by Dr Aseem Malholtra (Yellow Kite, 2021)
- *Authentic Happiness: Using the New Positive Psychology to Realise your Potential for Lasting Fulfilment* by Dr Martin Seligman (Nicholas Brealey Publishing, 2017)
- *Fat Chance: Beating the Odds Against Sugar, Processed Food, Obesity and Disease* by Dr Robert Lustig (Fourth Estate, 2014)
- *Forever Strong, A New Science-Based Strategy for Aging Well* by Dr Gabrielle Lyon (Piatkus, 2023)
- *Happy Relationships at Home, Work & Play* by Lucy Beresford (Prakash Book Depot, 2014)
- *Metabolical: The Truth About Processed Food and How It Poisons People and the Planet* by Dr Robert Lustig (Yellow Kite, 2021)
- *Oestrogen Matters: Why Taking Hormones in Menopause Can Improve Women's Well-Being and Lengthen Their Lives – Without Raising the Risk of Breast Cancer* by Dr Avrum Bluming and Carol Tavris (Piatkus, 2018)
- *Skin Food* by Dr Thivi Maruthappu (Piatkus, 2023)
- *Super Gut* by Dr William Davis (Yellow Kite, 2022)
- *The Big Fat Surprise: Why Butter, Meat and Cheese Belong in a Healthy Diet* by Nina Teicholz (Scribe UK, 2015)
- *The Definitive Guide to the Perimenopause and Menopause* by Dr Louise Newson (Yellow Kite, 2023)
- *The Diabetes Code: Prevent and Reverse Type 2 Diabetes Naturally* by Dr Jason Fung (Greystone Books, 2018)
- *The Five Minute Journal* (Intelligent Change, 2023)
- *The Harcombe Diet: Stop Counting Calories & Start Losing Weight* by Dr Zoë Harcombe (Columbus Publishing, 2020)

- *The Obesity Code: Unlocking the Secrets of Weight Loss* by Dr Jason Fung (Scribe UK, 2016)
- *The Pelvic Floor Bible: Everything You Need to Know to Prevent and Cure Problems at Every Stage in Your Life* by Jane Simpson (Penguin Life, 2019)
- *The Salt Fix: Why the Experts Got It All Wrong and How Eating More Might Save Your Life* by Dr James DiNicolantonio (Piatkus, 2017)
- *Therapeutic Fasting: The Buchinger Amplius Method* by Francoise Wilhelmi de Toledo (Thieme Medical Publishers, 2011)
- *The Top Five Regrets of the Dying* by Bronnie Ware (Hay House UK, 2019)
- *Ultra-Processed People: Why Do We All Eat Stuff That Isn't Food . . . and Why Can't We Stop?* by Chris van Tulleken (Cornerstone Press, 2023)

Suppliers

These are some of my favourite wellness suppliers. Many have generous LIZLOVES discount codes – see www.lizearlewellbeing.com/lizloves for current offers.

Coffee

Exhale: exhalecoffee.com
Specialising in high-polyphenol-content beans and blends.

Kingdom Coffee: kingdomcoffee.co.uk
Ethical and charity-focused coffee and tea supplier.

Rave: ravecoffee.co.uk
High-quality, extra-fresh coffees and blends.

Grounding

Bahé: bahe.co
For grounding trainers.

Get Grounded: getgrounded.co.uk
For grounding sheets and mats.

Herb teas

G. Baldwin & Co.: baldwins.co.uk

Herbal sleeping tinctures

Life Armour Slumber Drops: lifearmour.co.uk

Low-carb, zero-sugar and keto products

Anna's Keto Bakery: annasketobakery.co.uk
Delicious biscuits, muffins, breads as well as keto celebration cakes.

Hand Crafted Bread: handcraftedbread.co.uk
Award-winning range of breads, including sourdough and low-carb options

Lifeforce Organics: lifeforceorganics.co.uk
Organic and activated foods, such as nuts, seeds and wheat-free sourdough bread.

The Keto Bakery: theketobakery.com
Excellent keto brownies, granola, cakes, muffins and more.

WellEasy: welleasy.co.uk
One-stop shop for low-carb and keto breads, wraps, pasta, noodles and more, as well as many other wellbeing pantry staples.

Supplements
Adaptogens:
Karmacist: karmacist.com
Life Armour: lifearmour.co.uk

Bergamot:
Metabolic Gold, The Naked Pharmacy: thenakedpharmacy.com

Calm Complex:
BioCare: biocare.co.uk

Creatine: healf.com

CBD drops, oils, gummies and more:
Biogenic: biogeniccbd.co.uk

Electrolytes:
LMNT and Body Bio: both available from www.healf.com
True Hydration from Ancient & Brave: ancientandbrave.earth

Encapsulated collagen:
Ingenious Beauty: feelingenious.com

Fish oil:
Bare Biology: barebiology.com
Wild Nutrition: wildnutrition.com

Food-origin supplements:
Wild Nutrition: wildnutrition.com

Glutathione:
Youth & Earth: youthandearth.com

High phenolic olive oil:
The Governor: thegovernorevoo.co.uk

Kombucha drinks:
Liz Earle Wellbeing, Mighty Brew: mightybrew.com

Magnesium:
BetterYou: betteryou.com
Magnesium drink, Terranova: terranovahealth.com

MCT oil:
Ancient + Brave: ancientandbrave.earth

Medicinal mushrooms:
Bristol Fungarium: bristolfungarium.com

NAD+:
Nuchido: nuchido.com

NMN:
Youth & Earth: youthandearth.com

Nootropics:
Karmacist: karmacist.com

Omega-3:
Bare Biology: barebiology.com
Wild Nutrition: wildnutrition.com

Prebiotics
Bimuno: bimuno.com

Probiotics:
The Naked Pharmacy: thenakedpharmacy.com
Microbz: microbz.com
Quercetin
BioCare: biocare.co.uk

Resveratrol:
Youth & Earth: youthandearth.com

Seaweed:
Doctor Seaweed: doctorseaweed.com

Sleep drops and sprays:
Life Armour: lifearmour.co.uk
Better You: betteryou.com

Soil-based probiotics:
Microbz: microbz.co.uk

Spermidine:
Youth & Earth: youthandearth.com

Vitamin D3:
BetterYou: betteryou.com
The Naked Pharmacy: thenakedpharmacy.com

Weighted blankets
Aeyla: aeyla.co.uk

References

Ten Things I Wish I'd Known in My First Half

Li, S., Lear, S. A., Rangarajan, S., Hu, B., Yin, L., Bangdiwala, S. I., Alhabib, K. F., Rosengren, A., Gupta, R., Mony, P. K. and Wielgosz, A., 2022. Association of sitting time with mortality and cardiovascular events in high-income, middle-income, and low-income countries. *JAMA Cardiology*, 7(8), pp. 796–807.

Chapter 1: Prioritise You

Flossing
Boronow, K. E., Brody, J. G., Schaider, L. A., Peaslee, G. F., Havas, L. and Cohn, B. A., 2019. Serum concentrations of PFASs and exposure-related behaviors in African American and non-Hispanic white women. *Journal of Exposure Science and Environmental Epidemiology*, 29(2), pp. 206–17.

Goyal, C. R., Lyle, D. M., Qaqish, J. G. and Schuller, R., 2013. Evaluation of the plaque removal efficacy of a water flosser compared to string floss in adults after a single use. *Journal of Clinical Dentistry*, 24(2), pp. 37–42.

Get out, look up!
Taylor, D. N., Winfield, T. and Wynd, S., 2020. Low-level laser light therapy dosage variables vs treatment efficacy of neuromusculoskeletal conditions: A scoping review. *Journal of Chiropractic Medicine*, 19(2), pp. 119–27.

The benefits of 'grounding'
Oschman, J. L., Chevalier, G. and Brown, R., 2015. The effects of grounding (earthing) on inflammation, the immune response, wound healing, and prevention and treatment of chronic inflammatory and autoimmune diseases. *Journal of Inflammation Research*, pp. 83–96.

The gender divide
Lamvu, G., Antunez-Flores, O., Orady, M. and Schneider, B., 2020. Path to diagnosis and women's perspectives on the impact of endometriosis pain. *Journal of Endometriosis and Pelvic Pain Disorders*, *12*(1), pp. 16–25.

Le Louët, H. and Pitts, P. J., 2023. Twenty-first century global ADR management: A need for clarification, redesign, and coordinated action. *Therapeutic Innovation and Regulatory Science*, *57*(1), pp. 100–3.

Chapter 2: Reversing Ageing with Science

How to increase your odds with bio-hacking
Jing, H. and Lin, H., 2015. Sirtuins in epigenetic regulation. *Chemical Reviews*, *115*(6), pp. 2350–75.

Madeo, F., Carmona-Gutierrez, D., Kepp, O. and Kroemer, G., 2018. Spermidine delays aging in humans. *Aging* (Albany NY), *10*(8), p. 2209.

Autophagy and cancer prevention
Galluzzi, L., Pietrocola, F., Bravo-San Pedro, J. M., Amaravadi, R. K., Baehrecke, E. H., Cecconi, F., Codogno, P., Debnath, J., Gewirtz, D. A., Karantza, V. and Kimmelman, A., 2015. Autophagy in malignant transformation and cancer progression. *EMBO Journal*, *34*(7), pp. 856–80.

Hofer, S. J., Simon, A. K., Bergmann, M., Eisenberg, T., Kroemer, G. and Madeo, F., 2022. Mechanisms of spermidine-induced autophagy and geroprotection. *Nature Aging*, *2*(12), pp. 1112–29.

Co-enzyme Q10
Hargreaves, I. P., 2014. Coenzyme Q10 as a therapy for mitochondrial disease. *International Journal of Biochemistry and Cell Biology*, *49*, pp. 105–111.

Smith, K. M., Matson, S., Matson, W. R., Cormier, K., Del Signore, S. J., Hagerty, S. W., Stack, E. C., Ryu, H. and Ferrante, R. J., 2006. Dose ranging and efficacy study of high-dose coenzyme Q10 formulations in Huntington's disease mice. *Biochimica et Biophysica Acta (BBA)-Molecular Basis of Disease, 1762*(6), pp. 616–26.

Turunen, M., Olsson, J. and Dallner, G., 2004. Metabolism and function of coenzyme Q. *Biochimica et Biophysica Acta (BBA)-Biomembranes, 1660*(1–2), pp. 171–99.

Glutathione

Dilokthornsakul, W., Dhippayom, T. and Dilokthornsakul, P., 2019. The clinical effect of glutathione on skin color and other related skin conditions: A systematic review. *Journal of Cosmetic Dermatology, 18*(3), pp. 728–37.

Saxena, S., Gautam, R. K., Gupta, A. and Chitkara, A., 2020. Evaluation of systemic oxidative stress in patients with premature canities and correlation of severity of hair graying with the degree of redox imbalance. *International Journal of Trichology, 12*(1), p. 16.

Chapter 3: Hormone Hacking

Be guided by your symptoms

National Institute for Health and Care Excellence, 5 Dec. 2019. Menopause: Diagnosis and management. Retrieved from https://www.nice.org.uk/guidance/ng23 (accessed 29 Sep. 2023).

Common HRT myths

Akter, N., Kulinskaya, E., Steel, N. and Bakbergenuly, I., 2022. The effect of hormone replacement therapy on the survival of UK women: A retrospective cohort study 1984–2017. *BJOG: An International Journal of Obstetrics and Gynaecology, 129*(6), pp. 994–1003.

Bianchi, V. E., 2022. Impact of testosterone on Alzheimer's disease. *World Journal of Men's Health, 40*(2), p. 243.

Chlebowski, R. T., Anderson, G. L., Aragaki, A. K., Manson, J. E., Stefanick, M. L., Pan, K., Barrington, W., Kuller, L. H., Simon, M. S., Lane, D. and Johnson, K. C., 2020. Association of menopausal hormone therapy with breast cancer incidence and mortality during long-term follow-up of the women's health initiative randomized clinical trials. *JAMA, 324*(4), pp. 369–80.

Hodis, H. N. and Mack, W. J., 2022. Menopausal hormone replacement therapy and reduction of all-cause mortality and cardiovascular disease: It is about time and timing. *Cancer Journal, 28*(3), pp. 208–23.

Manson, J. E., Chlebowski, R. T., Stefanick, M. L., Aragaki, M. A. K., Rossouw, J. E., Prentice, R. L., Anderson, G., Howard, B. V., Thomson, C. A., LaCroix, A. Z. and Wactawski-Wende, J., 2013. The Women's Health Initiative hormone therapy trials: Update and overview of health outcomes during the intervention and post-stopping phases. *JAMA: the Journal of the American Medical Association, 310*(13), p. 1353.

Saleh, R. N., Hornberger, M., Ritchie, C. W. and Minihane, A. M., 2023. Hormone replacement therapy is associated with improved cognition and larger brain volumes in at-risk APOE4 women: Results from the European Prevention of Alzheimer's Disease (EPAD) cohort. *Alzheimer's Research and Therapy, 15*(1), p. 10.

HRT: What to expect

British Menopause Society, Mar. 2021. BMS & WHC's 2020 recommendations on hormone replacement therapy in menopausal women. Retrieved from https://thebms.org.uk/publications/consensus-statements/bms-whcs-2020-recommendations-on-hormone-replacement-therapy-in-menopausal-women/ (accessed 29 Sep. 2023).

Leopold, C. S. and Maibach, H. I., 1996. Effect of lipophilic vehicles on in vivo skin penetration of methyl nicotinate in different races. *International Journal Of Pharmaceutics, 139*(1–2), pp. 161–7.

Liu, P., Higuchi, W. I., Ghanem, A. H. and Good, W. R., 1994. Transport of β-estradiol in freshly excised human skin in vitro: Diffusion and metabolism in each skin layer. *Pharmaceutical Research, 11*, pp. 1777–84.

Newson Health, 9 Mar. 2023. HRT doses explained. Balance. Retrieved from https://www.balance-menopause.com/menopause-library/hrt-doses-explained/ (accessed 29 Sep. 2023).

Should all women take HRT?

Islam, R. M., Bell, R. J., Handelsman, D. J., McNeil, J. J., Nelson, M. R., Reid, C. M., Tonkin, A. M., Wolfe, R. S., Woods, R. L. and Davis, S. R., 2022.

Associations between blood sex steroid concentrations and risk of major adverse cardiovascular events in healthy older women in Australia: A prospective cohort substudy of the ASPREE trial. *Lancet Healthy Longevity*, *3*(2), pp. e109–18.

Mauvais-Jarvis, F., Manson, J. E., Stevenson, J. C. and Fonseca, V. A., 2017. Menopausal hormone therapy and type 2 diabetes prevention: Evidence, mechanisms, and clinical implications. *Endocrine Reviews*, *38*(3), pp. 173–88.

Nanda, K., Bastian, L. A., Hasselblad, V. and Simel, D. L., 1999. Hormone replacement therapy and the risk of colorectal cancer: A meta-analysis. *Obstetrics and Gynecology*, *93*(5), pp. 880–8.

The University of Arizona Health Sciences, 9 Jul. 2021. Researchers take a step toward advancing precision hormone therapies to reduce Alzheimer's risk. Retrieved from https://healthsciences.arizona.edu/newsroom/news-releases/2021/researchers-take-step-toward-advancing-precision-hormone-therapies#:~:text=A%20new%20University%20of%20Arizona,therapy%20and%20duration%20of%20use (accessed 29 Sep. 2023).

Herbs that can help in midlife

Booth, N. L., Piersen, C. E., Banuvar, S., Geller, S. E., Shulman, L. P. and Farnsworth, N. R., 2006. Clinical studies of red clover (Trifolium pratense) dietary supplements in menopause: A literature review. *Menopause*, *13*(2), pp. 251–64.

Kenda, M., Glavač, N. K., Nagy, M., Sollner Dolenc, M. and OEMONOM, 2021. Herbal products used in menopause and for gynecological disorders. *Molecules*, *26*(24), p. 7421.

Khapre, S., Deshmukh, U. and Jain, S., 2022. The impact of soy isoflavone supplementation on the menopausal symptoms in perimenopausal and postmenopausal women. *Journal of Mid-life Health*, *13*(2), p. 175.

Lethaby, A., Marjoribanks, J., Kronenberg, F., Roberts, H., Eden, J. and Brown, J., 2013. Phytoestrogens for menopausal vasomotor symptoms. *Cochrane Database of Systematic Reviews*, (12).

Nutrition for menopause

Ahad, F. and Ganie, S. A., 2010. Iodine, iodine metabolism and iodine deficiency disorders revisited. *Indian Journal of Endocrinology and Metabolism*, *14*(1), pp. 13–17.

Freeman, M. P., Hibbeln, J. R., Silver, M., Hirschberg, A. M., Wang, B., Yule, A. M., Petrillo, L. F., Pascuillo, E., Economou, N. I., Joffe, H. and Cohen, L. S., 2011. Omega-3 fatty acids for major depressive disorder associated with the menopausal transition: A preliminary open trial. *Menopause* (New York, NY), 18(3), p. 279.

Orchard, T. S., Larson, J. C., Alghothani, N., Bout-Tabaku, S., Cauley, J. A., Chen, Z., LaCroix, A. Z., Wactawski-Wende, J. and Jackson, R. D., 2014. Magnesium intake, bone mineral density, and fractures: Results from the Women's Health Initiative Observational Study. *American Journal of Clinical Nutrition, 99*(4), pp. 926–33.

Su, L. J., Chiang, T., and O'Connor, S. N., 2023. Arsenic in brown rice: do the benefits outwight the risks? *Frontiers in Nutrition.* Retrieved from https://www.ncbi.nlm.nih.gov/pmc/articles/PMC10375490/#:~:text=The%20investigation%20concluded%20that%20the,%27%20dry%2Dbrown%20rice%20cereal (accessed 28 Nov. 2023).

Sunyecz, J. A., 2008. The use of calcium and vitamin D in the management of osteoporosis. *Therapeutics and Clinical Risk Management, 4*(4), pp. 827–36.

Tarleton, E. K. and Littenberg, B., 2015. Magnesium intake and depression in adults. *Journal of the American Board of Family Medicine, 28*(2), pp. 249–56.

Wang, J., Um, P., Dickerman, B. A. and Liu, J., 2018. Zinc, magnesium, selenium and depression: A review of the evidence, potential mechanisms and implications. *Nutrients, 10*(5), p. 584.

Chapter 4: Eating to Age Well

The high-fat scandal

Seven Countries Study, n.d. About the study. Retrieved from https://www.sevencountriesstudy.com/about-the-study/ (accessed 29 Sep. 2023).

What about saturated fat?

Grasgruber, P., Sebera, M., Hrazdira, E., Hrebickova, S. and Cacek, J., 2016. Food consumption and the actual statistics of cardiovascular diseases: An epidemiological comparison of 42 European countries. *Food and Nutrition Research, 60*(1), p. 31694.

Praagman, J., Beulens, J. W., Alssema, M., Zock, P. L., Wanders, A. J., Sluijs, I. and Van Der Schouw, Y. T., 2016. The association between dietary saturated fatty acids and ischemic heart disease depends on the type and source of fatty acid in the European Prospective Investigation into Cancer and Nutrition–Netherlands cohort, 2. *American Journal of Clinical Nutrition, 103*(2), pp. 356–65.

Hydrogenated fats
Marchand, V., Canadian Paediatric Society and Nutrition and Gastroenterology Committee, 2010. Trans fats: What physicians should know. *Paediatrics and Child Health, 15*(6), pp. 373–5.

Spotlight on fats and oils
Allouche, Y., Jiménez, A., Gaforio, J. J., Uceda, M. and Beltrán, G., 2007. How heating affects extra virgin olive oil quality indexes and chemical composition. *Journal of Agricultural and Food Chemistry, 55*(23), pp. 9646–54.

Chiou, A. and Kalogeropoulos, N., 2017. Virgin olive oil as frying oil. *Comprehensive Reviews in Food Science and Food Safety, 16*(4), pp. 632–46.

Lands, W. E., 2005. Dietary fat and health: The evidence and the politics of prevention: Careful use of dietary fats can improve life and prevent disease. *Annals of the New York Academy of Sciences, 1055*(1), pp. 179–92.

Mazza, E., Fava, A., Ferro, Y., Rotundo, S., Romeo, S., Bosco, D., Pujia, A. and Montalcini, T., 2018. Effect of the replacement of dietary vegetable oils with a low dose of extra-virgin olive oil in the Mediterranean Diet on cognitive functions in the elderly. *Journal of Translational Medicine, 16*(1), pp. 1–10.

Omega 3-6
Innis, S. M., 2014. Omega-3 fatty acid biochemistry: Perspectives from human nutrition. *Military Medicine, 179*(suppl. 11), pp. 82–7.

Omega-9
Farag, M. A. and Gad, M. Z., 2022. Omega-9 fatty acids: Potential roles in inflammation and cancer management. *Journal of Genetic Engineering and Biotechnology, 20*(1), pp. 1–11.

Timing matters
Kubota, S., Liu, Y., Iizuka, K., Kuwata, H., Seino, Y. and Yabe, D., 2020. A review of recent findings on meal sequence: An attractive dietary approach to prevention and management of type 2 diabetes. *Nutrients*, *12*(9), p. 2502.

Why I changed my mind about meat
Brooks McCormick Jr Animal Law & Policy Program and Center for Environmental & Animal Protection, n.d. Animal markets and zoonotic disease in the United States. Harvard Law School. Retrieved from https://animal.law.harvard.edu/wp-content/uploads/Animal-Markets-and-Zoonotic-Disease-in-the-United-States.pdf (accessed 29 Sep. 2023).

The reality of junk food
Neumann, N. J. and Fasshauer, M., 2022. Added flavors: Potential contributors to body weight gain and obesity? *BMC Medicine*, *20*(1), p. 417.

Milk and dairy matters
Aslam, H., Marx, W., Rocks, T., Loughman, A., Chandrasekaran, V., Ruusunen, A., Dawson, S. L., West, M., Mullarkey, E., Pasco, J. A. and Jacka, F. N., 2020. The effects of dairy and dairy derivatives on the gut microbiota: A systematic literature review. *Gut Microbes*, *12*(1), p. 1799533.

Lordan, R., Tsoupras, A., Mitra, B. and Zabetakis, I., 2018. Dairy fats and cardiovascular disease: Do we really need to be concerned? *Foods*, *7*(3), p. 29.

A good egg
Matsuoka, R. and Sugano, M., 2022. Health functions of egg protein. *Foods*, *11*(15), p. 2309.

Ruff, K. J., Winkler, A., Jackson, R. W., DeVore, D. P. and Ritz, B. W., 2009. Eggshell membrane in the treatment of pain and stiffness from osteoarthritis of the knee: A randomized, multicenter, double-blind, placebo-controlled clinical study. *Clinical Rheumatology*, *28*, pp. 907–14.

Scholarly Community Encyclopedia, 10 Aug. 2022. Egg protein. Retrieved from https://encyclopedia.pub/entry/26002 (accessed 29 Sep. 2023).

Takanami Y., Kawai Y., Nakata C., Nishiyama H. and Matsuoka R. The combined effect of excise and lactic fermented egg white on the skeletal muscle function and muscle mass in middle-aged and elderly women. *In:* Tajima H., (ed.), 2015. *Proceedings of the 70th Annual Meeting of the Japanese Society of Physical Fitness and Sports Medicine, Wakayama, Japan, 18–20 September 2015.* The Japanese Society of Physical Fitness and Sports Medicine.

A fishy issue
Nøstbakken, O. J., Rasinger, J. D., Hannisdal, R., Sanden, M., Frøyland, L., Duinker, A., Frantzen, S., Dahl, L. M., Lundebye, A. K. and Madsen, L., 2021. Levels of omega 3 fatty acids, vitamin D, dioxins and dioxin-like PCBs in oily fish; a new perspective on the reporting of nutrient and contaminant data for risk–benefit assessments of oily seafood. *Environment International, 147*, p. 106322.

US Department of Veterans Affairs, n.d. VA's million veteran program publications through May 2022. Retrieved from https://www.mvp.va.gov/pwa/sites/default/files/2022-08/MVP%20Publications_2022-05.pdf (accessed 29 Sep. 2023).

Fruit and veg
Alavanja, M. C., 2009. Introduction: Pesticides use and exposure, extensive worldwide. *Reviews on Environmental Health, 24*(4), pp. 303–10.

Boffetta, P., Couto, E., Wichmann, J., Ferrari, P., Trichopoulos, D., Bueno-de-Mesquita, H. B., Van Duijnhoven, F. J., Büchner, F. L., Key, T., Boeing, H. and Nöthlings, U., 2010. Fruit and vegetable intake and overall cancer risk in the European Prospective Investigation into Cancer and Nutrition (EPIC). *Journal of the National Cancer Institute, 102*(8), pp. 529–37.

Hecht, S. S., Chung, F. L., Richie Jr, J. P., Akerkar, S. A., Borukhova, A., Skowronski, L. and Carmella, S. G., 1995. Effects of watercress consumption on metabolism of a tobacco-specific lung carcinogen in smokers. *Cancer Epidemiology, Biomarkers and Prevention: A Publication of the American Association for Cancer Research, Cosponsored by the American Society of Preventive Oncology, 4*(8), pp. 877–84.

Chocolate: Now for the good news!
Berk, L., Bruhjell, K., Peters, W., Bastian, P., Lohman, E., Bains, G., Arevalo, J. and Cole, S., 2018. Dark chocolate (70% cacao) effects human gene expression: Cacao regulates cellular immune response, neural signaling, and sensory perception. *FASEB Journal, 32*, p. 755.1.

Hooper, L., Kay, C., Abdelhamid, A., Kroon, P. A., Cohn, J. S., Rimm, E. B. and Cassidy, A., 2012. Effects of chocolate, cocoa, and flavan-3-ols on cardiovascular health: A systematic review and meta-analysis of randomized trials. *American Journal of Clinical Nutrition*, 95(3), pp. 740–51.

Jiménez, R., Duarte, J. and Perez-Vizcaino, F., 2012. Epicatechin: Endothelial function and blood pressure. *Journal of Agricultural and Food Chemistry*, 60(36), pp. 8823–30.

Rivas-Chacón, L. D. M., Yanes-Díaz, J., de Lucas, B., Riestra-Ayora, J. I., Madrid-García, R., Sanz-Fernández, R. and Sánchez-Rodríguez, C., 2023. Cocoa polyphenol extract inhibits cellular senescence via modulation of SIRT1 and SIRT3 in auditory cells. *Nutrients*, 15(3), p. 544.

Chapter 5: Maintaining a Healthy Weight in Midlife

Hall, K. D. and Kahan, S., 2018. Maintenance of lost weight and long-term management of obesity. *Medical Clinics*, 102(1), pp. 183–97.

Time-restricted eating for weight loss
Schuppelius, B., Peters, B., Ottawa, A. and Pivovarova-Ramich, O., 2021. Time restricted eating: A dietary strategy to prevent and treat metabolic disturbances. *Frontiers in Endocrinology*, 12, p. 683140.

Why sugar should be avoided
Mathur, K., Agrawal, R. K., Nagpure, S. and Deshpande, D., 2020. Effect of artificial sweeteners on insulin resistance among type-2 diabetes mellitus patients. *Journal of Family Medicine and Primary Care*, 9(1), p. 69.

Sugar substitutes
Choudhary, A. K. and Lee, Y. Y., 2018. Neurophysiological symptoms and aspartame: What is the connection? *Nutritional Neuroscience*, 21(5), pp. 306–16.

Liauw, S. and Saibil, F., 2019. Sorbitol: Often forgotten cause of osmotic diarrhea. *Canadian Family Physician*, 65(8), pp. 557–8.

National Institutes of Health, 14 Mar. 2023. Erythritol and cardiovascular events. Retrieved from https://www.nih.gov/news-events/nih-research-matters/erythritol-cardiovascular-events#:~:text=For%20at%20least%20two%20days,of%20heart%20attack%20or%20stroke (accessed 29 Sep. 2023).

Nayak, P. A., Nayak, U. A. and Khandelwal, V., 2014. The effect of xylitol on dental caries and oral flora. *Clinical, Cosmetic and Investigational Dentistry*, pp. 89–94.

O'Mary, L., 1 Jun. 2023. Sucralose damages DNA, linked to leaky gut: Study. WebMD. Retrieved from https://www.medscape.com/viewarticle/992667?ecd=mkm_ret_230607_mscpmrk-OUS_ICYMI&uac=456512PN&impID=5499758&faf=1 (accessed 29 Sep. 2023).

Schiffman, S. S., Scholl, E. H., Furey, T. S. and Nagle, H. T., 2023. Toxicological and pharmacokinetic properties of sucralose-6-acetate and its parent sucralose: in vitro screening assays. *Journal of Toxicology and Environmental Health, Part B*, pp. 1–35.

Science, 3 Nov, 1997. Saccharin: Still potentially dangerous. Retrieved from https://www.science.org/content/article/saccharin-still-potentially-dangerous (accessed 29 Sep. 2023).

Witkowski, M., Nemet, I., Alamri, H., Wilcox, J., Gupta, N., Nimer, N., Haghikia, A., Li, X.S., Wu, Y., Saha, P. P. and Demuth, I., 2023. The artificial sweetener erythritol and cardiovascular event risk. *Nature Medicine*, 29(3), pp. 710–18.

Zhou, Y., Zheng, Y., Ebersole, J. and Huang, C. F., 2009. Insulin secretion stimulating effects of mogroside V and fruit extract of luo han kuo (Siraitia grosvenori Swingle) fruit extract. *Yao xue xue bao= Acta pharmaceutica Sinica*, 44(11), pp. 1252–7.

Supplements to support weight loss

Demura, S., Yamada, T., Yamaji, S., Komatsu, M. and Morishita, K., 2010. The effect of L-ornithine hydrochloride ingestion on human growth hormone secretion after strength training. *Advances in Bioscience and Biotechnology*, 1(01), pp. 7–11.

Dulloo, A. G., Duret, C., Rohrer, D., Girardier, L., Mensi, N., Fathi, M., Chantre, P. and Vandermander, J., 1999. Efficacy of a green tea extract rich in catechin polyphenols and caffeine in increasing 24-h energy expenditure and fat oxidation in humans. *American Journal of Clinical Nutrition*, 70(6), pp. 1040–5.

Glick, D., Barth, S. and Macleod, K. F., 2010. Autophagy: Cellular and molecular mechanisms. *Journal of Pathology*, 221(1), pp. 3–12.

Guo, H. H., Shen, H. R., Wang, L. L., Luo, Z. G., Zhang, J. L., Zhang, H. J., Gao, T. L., Han, Y. X. and Jiang, J. D., 2023. Berberine is a potential alternative for metformin with good regulatory effect on lipids in treating metabolic diseases. *Biomedicine and Pharmacotherapy*, 163, p. 114754.

Kiechl, S., Pechlaner, R., Willeit, P., Notdurfter, M., Paulweber, B., Willeit, K., Werner, P., Ruckenstuhl, C., Iglseder, B., Weger, S. and Mairhofer, B., 2018. Higher spermidine intake is linked to lower mortality: A prospective population-based study. *American Journal of Clinical Nutrition*, 108(2), pp. 371–80.

Madeo, F., Eisenberg, T., Pietrocola, F. and Kroemer, G., 2018. Spermidine in health and disease. *Science*, 359(6374), p. eaan2788.

Park, H. J., Jung, E. and Shim, I., 2020. Berberine for appetite suppressant and prevention of obesity. *BioMed Research International* retrieved from https://www.ncbi.nlm.nih.gov/pmc/articles/PMC7752296 (accessed 10 Jan. 2024).

Perna, S., Spadaccini, D., Botteri, L., Girometta, C., Riva, A., Allegrini, P., Petrangolini, G., Infantino, V. and Rondanelli, M., 2019. Efficacy of bergamot: From anti-inflammatory and anti-oxidative mechanisms to clinical applications as preventive agent for cardiovascular morbidity, skin diseases, and mood alterations. *Food Science and Nutrition*, 7(2), pp. 369–84.

Venables, M. C., Hulston, C. J., Cox, H. R. and Jeukendrup, A. E., 2008. Green tea extract ingestion, fat oxidation, and glucose tolerance in healthy humans. *American Journal of Clinical Nutrition*, 87(3), pp. 778–84.

Zhang, Y., Yu, Y., Li, X., Meguro, S., Hayashi, S., Katashima, M., Yasumasu, T., Wang, J. and Li, K., 2012. Effects of catechin-enriched green tea beverage on visceral fat loss in adults with a high proportion of visceral fat: A double-blind, placebo-controlled, randomized trial. *Journal of Functional Foods*, 4(1), pp. 315–22.

Birketvedt, G. S., Shimshi, M., Erling, T. and Florholmen, J., 2005. Experiences with three different fiber supplements in weight reduction. *Medical Science Monitor*, 11(1), pp. 15–18.

Chapter 6: You Are What You Drink

How electrolytes support our health

Latzka, W. A. and Montain, S. J., 1999. Water and electrolyte requirements for exercise. *Clinics in Sports Medicine, 18*(3), pp. 513–24.

Maughan, R. J. and Shirreffs, S. M., 2010. Development of hydration strategies to optimize performance for athletes in high-intensity sports and in sports with repeated intense efforts. *Scandinavian Journal of Medicine and Science in Sports, 20*, pp. 59–69.

Shirreffs, S. M. and Sawka, M. N., 2011. Fluid and electrolyte needs for training, competition, and recovery. *Journal of Sports Sciences, 29*(suppl. 1), pp. S39–46.

The case for more coffee

Antipolis, S., 27 Sep. 2022. Coffee drinking is associated with increased longevity. European Society of Cardiology. Retrieved from https://www.escardio.org/The-ESC/Press-Office/Press-releases/Coffee-drinking-is-associated-with-increased-longevity (accessed 29 Sep. 2023).

Harvard T. H. Chan School of Public Health, Jul. 2020. Coffee. Retrieved from https://www.hsph.harvard.edu/nutritionsource/food-features/coffee/ (accessed 29 Sep. 2023).

Liu, J. J., Crous-Bou, M., Giovannucci, E. and De Vivo, I., 2016. Coffee consumption is positively associated with longer leukocyte telomere length in the nurses' health study. *Journal of Nutrition, 146*(7), pp. 1373–8.

Poole, R., Kennedy, O. J., Roderick, P., Fallowfield, J. A., Hayes, P. C. and Parkes, J., 2017. Coffee consumption and health: Umbrella review of meta-analyses of multiple health outcomes. *BMJ, 359*. Retrieved from https://www.bmj.com/content/359/bmj.j5024 (accessed 10 Jan. 2024).

Tucker, L. A., 2017. Caffeine consumption and telomere length in men and women of the National Health and Nutrition Examination Survey (NHANES). *Nutrition and Metabolism, 14*(1), pp. 1–10.

Mould and mycotoxins explained

García-Moraleja, A., Font, G., Mañes, J. and Ferrer, E., 2015. Analysis of mycotoxins in coffee and risk assessment in Spanish adolescents and adults. *Food and Chemical Toxicology, 86*, pp. 225–33.

Sachdev, P. and Hogan, L., 24 Nov. 2021. What are mycotoxins? WebMD. Retrieved from https://www.webmd.com/food-recipes/food-poisoning/what-are-mycotoxins (accessed 31 Jan. 2023).

The health benefits of tea

Antipolis, S., 9 Jan. 2019. Tea drinkers live longer. European Society of Cardiology. Retrieved from https://www.escardio.org/The-ESC/Press-Office/Press-releases/Tea-drinkers-live-longer#:~:text=Compared%20with%20never%20or%20non,risk%20of%20all%2Dcause%20death (accessed 29 Sep. 2023).

Kumar Singh, A., Cabral, C., Kumar, R., Ganguly, R., Kumar Rana, H., Gupta, A., Rosaria Lauro, M., Carbone, C., Reis, F. and Pandey, A. K., 2019. Beneficial effects of dietary polyphenols on gut microbiota and strategies to improve delivery efficiency. *Nutrients*, *11*(9), p. 2216.

Kyle, J. A., Morrice, P. C., McNeill, G. and Duthie, G. G., 2007. Effects of infusion time and addition of milk on content and absorption of polyphenols from black tea. *Journal of Agricultural and Food Chemistry*, *55*(12), pp. 4889–94.

Williams, J. L., Everett, J. M., D'Cunha, N. M., Sergi, D., Georgousopoulou, E. N., Keegan, R. J., McKune, A. J., Mellor, D. D., Anstice, N. and Naumovski, N., 2020. The effects of green tea amino acid L-theanine consumption on the ability to manage stress and anxiety levels: A systematic review. *Plant Foods for Human Nutrition*, *75*, pp. 12–23.

Yan, Z., Zhong, Y., Duan, Y., Chen, Q. and Li, F., 2020. Antioxidant mechanism of tea polyphenols and its impact on health benefits. *Animal Nutrition*, *6*(2), pp. 115–23.

Herb teas

Adib-Hajbaghery, M. and Mousavi, S. N., 2017. The effects of chamomile extract on sleep quality among elderly people: A clinical trial. *Complementary Therapies in Medicine*, *35*, pp. 109–14.

Azevedo, M. F., Lima, C. F., Fernandes-Ferreira, M., Almeida, M. J., Wilson, J. M. and Pereira-Wilson, C., 2011. Rosmarinic acid, major phenolic constituent of Greek sage herbal tea, modulates rat intestinal SGLT1 levels with effects on blood glucose. *Molecular Nutrition and Food Research*, *55*(S1), pp. S15–25.

Cases, J., Ibarra, A., Feuillère, N., Roller, M. and Sukkar, S. G., 2011. Pilot trial of Melissa officinalis L. leaf extract in the treatment of volunteers suffering from mild-to-moderate anxiety disorders and sleep disturbances. *Mediterranean Journal of Nutrition and Metabolism, 4*(3), pp. 211–18.

Dludla, P. V., Joubert, E., Muller, C. J., Louw, J. and Johnson, R., 2017. Hyperglycemia-induced oxidative stress and heart disease-cardioprotective effects of rooibos flavonoids and phenylpyruvic acid-2-O-β-D-glucoside. *Nutrition and Metabolism, 14*(1), pp. 1–18.

Ebrahimzadeh, A., Ebrahimzadeh, A., Mirghazanfari, S. M., Hazrati, E., Hadi, S. and Milajerdi, A., 2022. The effect of ginger supplementation on metabolic profiles in patients with type 2 diabetes mellitus: A systematic review and meta-analysis of randomized controlled trials. *Complementary Therapies in Medicine, 65*, p. 102802.

Ellis, L. R., Zulfiqar, S., Holmes, M., Marshall, L., Dye, L. and Boesch, C., 2022. A systematic review and meta-analysis of the effects of Hibiscus sabdariffa on blood pressure and cardiometabolic markers. *Nutrition Reviews, 80*(6), pp. 1723–37.

Ghazizadeh, J., Sadigh-Eteghad, S., Marx, W., Fakhari, A., Hamedeyazdan, S., Torbati, M., Taheri-Tarighi, S., Araj-khodaei, M. and Mirghafourvand, M., 2021. The effects of lemon balm (Melissa officinalis L.) on depression and anxiety in clinical trials: A systematic review and meta-analysis. *Phytotherapy Research, 35*(12), pp. 6690–705.

Hocaoglu, A. B., Karaman, O., Erge, D. O., Erbil, G., Yilmaz, O., Bagriyanik, A. and Uzuner, N., 2011. Glycyrrhizin and long-term histopathologic changes in a murine model of asthma. *Current Therapeutic Research, 72*(6), pp. 250–61.

Ingrosso, M. R., Ianiro, G., Nee, J., Lembo, A. J., Moayyedi, P., Black, C. J. and Ford, A. C., 2022. Systematic review and meta-analysis: efficacy of peppermint oil in irritable bowel syndrome. *Alimentary Pharmacology and Therapeutics, 56*(6), pp. 932–41.

Khanna, R., MacDonald, J. K. and Levesque, B. G., 2014. Peppermint oil for the treatment of irritable bowel syndrome: A systematic review and meta-analysis. *Journal of Clinical Gastroenterology, 48*(6), pp. 505–12.

Mao, Q. Q., Xu, X. Y., Cao, S. Y., Gan, R. Y., Corke, H., Beta, T. and Li, H. B., 2019. Bioactive compounds and bioactivities of ginger (Zingiber officinale Roscoe). *Foods, 8*(6), p. 185.

Mollabashi, E. N., Ziaie, T. and Khalesi, Z. B., 2021. The effect of Matricaria chamomile on menstrual related mood disorders. *European Journal of Obstetrics and Gynecology and Reproductive Biology: X, 12*, p. 100134.

Icahn School of Medicine at Mount Sinai, 2023. Licorice. Retrieved from https://www.mountsinai.org/health-library/herb/licorice (accessed 29 Sep. 2023).

ScienceDirect, n.d. Lemon balm: An overview. Retrieved from https://www.sciencedirect.com/topics/agricultural-and-biological-sciences/lemon-balm (accessed 29 Sep. 2023).

Walch, S. G., Tinzoh, L. N., Zimmermann, B. F., Stühlinger, W. and Lachenmeier, D. W., 2011. Antioxidant capacity and polyphenolic composition as quality indicators for aqueous infusions of Salvia officinalis L.(sage tea). *Frontiers in Pharmacology*, 2, p. 79.

Wang, L., Yang, R., Yuan, B., Liu, Y. and Liu, C., 2015. The antiviral and antimicrobial activities of licorice, a widely-used Chinese herb. *Acta Pharmaceutica Sinica B*, 5(4), pp. 310–15.

Wightman, E. L., Jackson, P. A., Spittlehouse, B., Heffernan, T., Guillemet, D. and Kennedy, D. O., 2021. The acute and chronic cognitive effects of a sage extract: a randomized, placebo controlled study in healthy humans. *Nutrients*, 13(1), p. 218.

Yehuda, I., Madar, Z., Leikin-Frenkel, A. and Tamir, S., 2015. Glabridin, an isoflavan from licorice root, downregulates iNOS expression and activity under high-glucose stress and inflammation. *Molecular Nutrition and Food Research*, 59(6), pp. 1041–52.

Zemestani, M., Rafraf, M. and Asghari-Jafarabadi, M., 2016. Chamomile tea improves glycemic indices and antioxidants status in patients with type 2 diabetes mellitus. *Nutrition*, 32(1), pp. 66–72.

Zhang, B., Yue, R., Wang, Y., Wang, L., Chin, J., Huang, X. and Jiang, Y., 2020. Effect of Hibiscus sabdariffa (Roselle) supplementation in regulating blood lipids among patients with metabolic syndrome and related disorders: A systematic review and meta-analysis. *Phytotherapy Research*, 34(5), pp. 1083–95.

The 'demon' drink

Bertelli, A. A. and Das, D. K., 2009. Grapes, wines, resveratrol, and heart health. *Journal of Cardiovascular Pharmacology*, 54(6), pp. 468–76.

Facchini, F., Ida Chen, Y. D. and Reaven, G. M., 1994. Light-to-moderate alcohol intake is associated with enhanced insulin sensitivity. *Diabetes Care*, 17(2), pp. 115–19.

Micallef, M., Lexis, L. and Lewandowski, P., 2007. Red wine consumption increases antioxidant status and decreases oxidative stress in the circulation of both young and old humans. *Nutrition Journal*, *6*(1), pp. 1–8.

Mukamal, K. J., Kuller, L. H., Fitzpatrick, A. L., Longstreth Jr, W. T., Mittleman, M. A. and Siscovick, D. S., 2003. Prospective study of alcohol consumption and risk of dementia in older adults. *JAMA*, *289*(11), pp. 1405–13.

Salehi, B., Mishra, A. P., Nigam, M., Sener, B., Kilic, M., Sharifi-Rad, M., Fokou, P. V. T., Martins, N. and Sharifi-Rad, J., 2018. Resveratrol: A double-edged sword in health benefits. *Biomedicines*, *6*(3), p. 91.

Wood, A. M., Kaptoge, S., Butterworth, A. S., Willeit, P., Warnakula, S., Bolton, T., Paige, E., Paul, D. S., Sweeting, M., Burgess, S. and Bell, S., 2018. Risk thresholds for alcohol consumption: Combined analysis of individual-participant data for 599 912 current drinkers in 83 prospective studies. *Lancet*, *391*(10129), pp. 1513–23.

Chapter 7: Healthy Ageing Lies in Your Gut Health

Dabos, K. J., Sfika, E., Vlatta, L. J. and Giannikopoulos, G., 2010. The effect of mastic gum on Helicobacter pylori: A randomized pilot study. *Phytomedicine*, *17*(3–4), pp. 296–9.

Fernández-Murga, M. L., Gil-Ortiz, F., Serrano-García, L. and Llombart-Cussac, A., 2023. A new paradigm in the relationship between gut microbiota and breast cancer: β-glucuronidase enzyme identified as potential therapeutic target. *Pathogens*, *12*(9), p. 1086.

Fu, J., Bonder, M. J., Cenit, M. C., Tigchelaar, E. F., Maatman, A., Dekens, J. A., Brandsma, E., Marczynska, J., Imhann, F., Weersma, R. K. and Franke, L., 2015. The gut microbiome contributes to a substantial proportion of the variation in blood lipids. *Circulation Research*, *117*(9), pp. 817–24.

Han, N., Jia, L., Su, Y., Du, J., Guo, L., Luo, Z. and Liu, Y., 2019. Lactobacillus reuteri extracts promoted wound healing via PI3K/AKT/β-catenin/TGFβ1 pathway. *Stem Cell Research and Therapy*, *10*, pp. 1–11.

He, S., Li, H., Yu, Z., Zhang, F., Liang, S., Liu, H., Chen, H. and Lü, M., 2021. The gut microbiome and sex hormone-related diseases. *Frontiers in Microbiology*, p. 2699.

Masoumi, S. J., Mehrabani, D., Saberifiroozi, M., Fattahi, M. R., Moradi, F. and Najafi, M., 2021. The effect of yogurt fortified with Lactobacillus acidophilus and Bifidobacterium sp. probiotic in patients with lactose intolerance. *Food Science and Nutrition, 9*(3), pp. 1704–11.

Mohammadi, A. A., Jazayeri, S., Khosravi-Darani, K., Solati, Z., Mohammadpour, N., Asemi, Z., Adab, Z., Djalali, M., Tehrani-Doost, M., Hosseini, M. and Eghtesadi, S., 2016. The effects of probiotics on mental health and hypothalamic–pituitary–adrenal axis: A randomized, double-blind, placebo-controlled trial in petrochemical workers. *Nutritional Neuroscience, 19*(9), pp. 387–95.

Pinto-Sanchez, M. I., Hall, G. B., Ghajar, K., Nardelli, A., Bolino, C., Lau, J. T., Martin, F. P., Cominetti, O., Welsh, C., Rieder, A. and Traynor, J., 2017. Probiotic Bifidobacterium longum NCC3001 reduces depression scores and alters brain activity: A pilot study in patients with irritable bowel syndrome. *Gastroenterology, 153*(2), pp. 448–59.

Ridaura, V. K., Faith, J. J., Rey, F. E., Cheng, J., Duncan, A. E., Kau, A. L., Griffin, N. W., Lombard, V., Henrissat, B., Bain, J. R. and Muehlbauer, M. J., 2013. Gut microbiota from twins discordant for obesity modulate metabolism in mice. *Science, 341*(6150), p. 1241214.

ScienceDirect, n.d. Lactobacillus reuteri. Retrieved from https://www.sciencedirect.com/topics/agricultural-and-biological-sciences/lactobacillus-reuteri#:~:text=Strains%20are%20isolated%20from%20dairy,%2C%20Roncal%2C%20and%20Toma) (accessed 29 Sep. 2023).

Tagliari, E., Campos, L. F., Campos, A. C., Costa-Casagrande, T. A. and Noronha, L. D., 2019. Effect of probiotic oral administration on skin wound healing in rats. *ABCD. Arquivos Brasileiros de Cirurgia Digestiva (São Paulo), 32.*

Yousefnejad, H., Mohammadi, F., Alizadeh-Naini, M. and Hejazi, N., 2023. Nigella sativa powder for helicobacter pylori infected patients: A randomized, double-blinded, placebo-controlled clinical trial. *BMC Complementary Medicine and Therapies, 23*(1), pp. 1–7.

Probiotics

Metagenics, n.d. Probiotic strains for immune and gut wellbeing [infographic]. Retrieved from https://www.metagenicsinstitute.com.au/static-assets/content/pdfs/probiotics/Probiotic%20Infographic.pdf (accessed 29 Sep. 2023).

Sanders, M. E. and Klaenhammer, T. R., 2001. Invited review: The scientific basis of Lactobacillus acidophilus NCFM functionality as a probiotic. *Journal of Dairy Science, 84*(2), pp. 319–31.

Postbiotics

Moroi, M., Uchi, S., Nakamura, K., Sato, S., Shimizu, N., Fujii, M., Kumagai, T., Saito, M., Uchiyama, K., Watanabe, T. and Yamaguchi, H., 2011. Beneficial effect of a diet containing heat-killed Lactobacillus paracasei K71 on adult type atopic dermatitis. *Journal of Dermatology, 38*(2), pp. 131–9.

Sabatino, A. D., Morera, R., Ciccocioppo, R., Cazzola, P., Gotti, S., Tinozzi, F. P., Tinozzi, S. and Corazza, G. R., 2005. Oral butyrate for mildly to moderately active Crohn's disease. *Alimentary Pharmacology and Therapeutics, 22*(9), pp. 789–94.

Kamut

Hosie, R., 1 Oct. 2018. 75% of supermarket sourdough breads don't follow authentic recipe. *Independent*. Retrieved from https://www.independent.co.uk/life-style/food-and-drink/bread-to-buy-sourdough-best-where-real-extra-other-ingredients-recipe-a8563661.html# (accessed 29 Sep. 2023).

Lau, S. W., Chong, A. Q., Chin, N. L., Talib, R. A. and Basha, R. K., 2021. Sourdough microbiome comparison and benefits. *Microorganisms, 9*(7), p. 1355.

Kefir

Leite, A. M. D. O., Miguel, M. A. L., Peixoto, R. S., Rosado, A. S., Silva, J. T. and Paschoalin, V. M. F., 2013. Microbiological, technological and therapeutic properties of kefir: A natural probiotic beverage. *Brazilian Journal of Microbiology, 44*, pp. 341–9.

Kimchi

Seo, H., Bae, J. H., Kim, G., Kim, S. A., Ryu, B. H. and Han, N. S., 2021. Suitability analysis of 17 probiotic type strains of lactic acid bacteria as starter for kimchi fermentation. *Foods, 10*(6), p. 1435.

Kombucha

Yang, J., Lagishetty, V., Kurnia, P., Henning, S. M., Ahdoot, A. I. and Jacobs, J. P., 2022. Microbial and chemical profiles of commercial kombucha products. *Nutrients*, 14(3), p. 670.

Kraut

Zabat, M. A., Sano, W. H., Wurster, J. I., Cabral, D. J. and Belenky, P., 2018. Microbial community analysis of sauerkraut fermentation reveals a stable and rapidly established community. *Foods*, 7(5), p. 77.

Cacao

Sorrenti, V., Ali, S., Mancin, L., Davinelli, S., Paoli, A. and Scapagnini, G., 2020. Cocoa polyphenols and gut microbiota interplay: Bioavailability, prebiotic effect, and impact on human health. *Nutrients*, 12(7), p. 1908.

When *not* to eat

Zeb, F., Osaili, T., Obaid, R. S., Naja, F., Radwan, H., Cheikh Ismail, L., Hasan, H., Hashim, M., Alam, I., Sehar, B. and Faris, M. E., 2023. Gut microbiota and time-restricted feeding/eating: A targeted biomarker and approach in precision nutrition. *Nutrients*, 15(2), p. 259.

Apple cider vinegar

Hadi, A., Pourmasoumi, M., Najafgholizadeh, A., Clark, C. C. and Esmaillzadeh, A., 2021. The effect of apple cider vinegar on lipid profiles and glycemic parameters: A systematic review and meta-analysis of randomized clinical trials. *BMC Complementary Medicine and Therapies*, 21(1), p. 179.

Olive leaf extract

Barbaro, B., Toietta, G., Maggio, R., Arciello, M., Tarocchi, M., Galli, A. and Balsano, C., 2014. Effects of the olive-derived polyphenol oleuropein on human health. *International Journal of Molecular Sciences*, 15(10), pp. 18508–24.

Vogel, P., Machado, I. K., Garavaglia, J., Zani, V. T., de Souza, D. and Dal Bosco, S. M., 2015. Polyphenols benefits of olive leaf (Olea europaea L) to human health. *Nutrición Hospitalaria*, 31(3), pp. 1427–33.

Zhu, M., Liu, X., Ye, Y., Yan, X., Cheng, Y., Zhao, L., Chen, F. and Ling, Z., 2022. Gut microbiota: A novel therapeutic target for Parkinson's disease. *Frontiers in Immunology, 13*, p. 937555.

Slippery elm

Ahuja, A. and Ahuja, N. K., 2019. Popular remedies for esophageal symptoms: A critical appraisal. *Current Gastroenterology Reports, 21*, pp. 1–8.

Hawrelak, J. A. and Myers, S. P., 2010. Effects of two natural medicine formulations on irritable bowel syndrome symptoms: A pilot study. *The Journal of Alternative and Complementary Medicine, 16*(10), pp. 1065–71.

Langmead, L., Dawson, C., Hawkins, C., Banna, N., Loo, S. and Rampton, D. S., 2002. Antioxidant effects of herbal therapies used by patients with inflammatory bowel disease: An in vitro study. *Alimentary Pharmacology and Therapeutics, 16*(2), pp. 197–205.

Ried, K., Travica, N., Dorairaj, R. and Sali, A., 2020. Herbal formula improves upper and lower gastrointestinal symptoms and gut health in Australian adults with digestive disorders. *Nutrition Research, 76*, pp. 37–51.

Whey

Benjamin, J., Makharia, G., Ahuja, V., Anand Rajan, K. D., Kalaivani, M., Gupta, S. D. and Joshi, Y. K., 2012. Glutamine and whey protein improve intestinal permeability and morphology in patients with Crohn's disease: A randomized controlled trial. *Digestive Diseases and Sciences, 57*, pp. 1000–12.

Pal, S. and Ellis, V., 2010. The chronic effects of whey proteins on blood pressure, vascular function, and inflammatory markers in overweight individuals. *Obesity, 18*(7), pp. 1354–9.

Chapter 8: Protecting the Brain

Why fish fats are key

Heude, B., Ducimetière, P. and Berr, C., 2003. Cognitive decline and fatty acid composition of erythrocyte membranes – The EVA Study. *American Journal of Clinical Nutrition, 77*(4), pp. 803–8.

Lee, L. K., Shahar, S., Chin, A. V. and Yusoff, N. A. M., 2013. Docosahexaenoic acid-concentrated fish oil supplementation in subjects with mild cognitive impairment (MCI): A 12-month randomised, double-blind, placebo-controlled trial. *Psychopharmacology*, 225, pp. 605–12.

Lukaschek, K., Von Schacky, C., Kruse, J. and Ladwig, K. H., 2016. Cognitive impairment is associated with a low omega-3 index in the elderly: Results from the KORA-Age study. *Dementia and Geriatric Cognitive Disorders*, 42(3–4), pp. 236–45.

Schaefer, E. J., Bongard, V., Beiser, A. S., Lamon-Fava, S., Robins, S. J., Au, R., Tucker, K. L., Kyle, D. J., Wilson, P. W. and Wolf, P. A., 2006. Plasma phosphatidylcholine docosahexaenoic acid content and risk of dementia and Alzheimer disease: The Framingham Heart Study. *Archives of Neurology*, 63(11), pp. 1545–50.

Thomas, A., Crivello, F., Mazoyer, B., Debette, S., Tzourio, C. and Samieri, C., 2021. Fish intake and MRI burden of cerebrovascular disease in older adults. *Neurology*, 97(22), pp. e2213–22.

Yurko-Mauro, K., Kralovec, J., Bailey-Hall, E., Smeberg, V., Stark, J. G. and Salem, N., 2015. Similar eicosapentaenoic acid and docosahexaenoic acid plasma levels achieved with fish oil or krill oil in a randomized double-blind four-week bioavailability study. *Lipids in Health and Disease*, 14, pp. 1–9.

Brain boosters

Kennedy, D. O., Haskell, C. F., Mauri, P. L. and Scholey, A. B., 2007. Acute cognitive effects of standardised Ginkgo biloba extract complexed with phosphatidylserine. *Human Psychopharmacology: Clinical and Experimental*, 22(4), pp. 199–210.

Nash, K. M., and Shah, Z. A., 2015. Current perspectives on the beneficial role of Ginkgo biloba in neurological and cerebrovascular disorders. *Integrative Medicine Insights*, 10, pp. 1–9.

Zuo, W., Yan, F., Zhang, B., Li, J. and Mei, D., 2017. Advances in the studies of Ginkgo biloba leaves extract on aging-related diseases. *Aging and Disease*, 8(6), p. 812.

Chaga

Eley, E., 23 Jun. 2011. Chaga mushrooms could aid memory loss and other cognitive functions [blog]. Royal Society of Chemistry. Retrieved from https://blogs.rsc.org/fo/2011/06/23/chaga-mushrooms-could-aid-memory-loss-and-other-cognitive-functions/?doing_wp_cron=1687612598.679765939 7125244140625 (accessed 29 Sep. 2023).

Cordyceps
Zhang, X., Wang, M., Qiao, Y., Shan, Z., Yang, M., Li, G., Xiao, Y., Wei, L., Bi, H. and Gao, T., 2022. Exploring the mechanisms of action of Cordyceps sinensis for the treatment of depression using network pharmacology and molecular docking. *Annals of Translational Medicine, 10*(6).

Lion's mane
Lai, P. L., Naidu, M., Sabaratnam, V., Wong, K. H., David, R. P., Kuppusamy, U. R., Abdullah, N. and Malek, S. N. A., 2013. Neurotrophic properties of the Lion's mane medicinal mushroom, Hericium erinaceus (Higher Basidiomycetes) from Malaysia. *International Journal of Medicinal Mushrooms, 15*(6).

Maitake
Bao, H., Ran, P., Sun, L., Hu, W., Li, H., Xiao, C., Zhu, K. and Du, J., 2017. Griflola frondosa (GF) produces significant antidepressant effects involving AMPA receptor activation in mice. *Pharmaceutical Biology, 55*(1), pp. 299–305.

Reishi
Wachtel-Galor, S., Tomlinson, B. and Benzie, I. F., 2004. Ganoderma lucidum ('Lingzhi'), a Chinese medicinal mushroom: Biomarker responses in a controlled human supplementation study. *British Journal of Nutrition, 91*(2), pp. 263–9.

Zhao, H., Zhang, Q., Zhao, L., Huang, X., Wang, J. and Kang, X., 2012. Spore powder of Ganoderma lucidum improves cancer-related fatigue in breast cancer patients undergoing endocrine therapy: A pilot clinical trial. *Evidence-Based Complementary and Alternative Medicine.*

Shiitake
Aldwinckle, J. and Kristiansen, B., 2020. A Quality-of-life study in healthy adults supplemented with Lentinex® beta-glucan of shiitake culinary – medicinal mushroom, lentinus edodes (agaricomycetes). *International Journal of Medicinal Mushrooms, 22*(5).

Dai, X., Stanilka, J. M., Rowe, C. A., Esteves, E. A., Nieves Jr, C., Spaiser, S. J., Christman, M. C., Langkamp-Henken, B. and Percival, S. S., 2015. Consuming Lentinula edodes (Shiitake) mushrooms daily improves human immunity: A randomized dietary intervention in healthy young adults. *Journal of the American College of Nutrition, 34*(6), pp. 478–87.

Finimundy, T. C., Dillon, A. J. P., Henriques, J. A. P. and Ely, M. R., 2014. A review on general nutritional compounds and pharmacological properties of the Lentinula edodes mushroom. *Food and Nutrition Sciences.*

Turkey tail
Guggenheim, A. G., Wright, K. M. and Zwickey, H. L., 2014. Immune modulation from five major mushrooms: Application to integrative oncology. *Integrative Medicine: A Clinician's Journal, 13*(1), p. 32.

Ma, Y., Wu, X., Yu, J., Zhu, J., Pen, X. and Meng, X., 2017. Can polysaccharide K improve therapeutic efficacy and safety in gastrointestinal cancer? A systematic review and network meta-analysis. *Oncotarget, 8*(51), p. 89108.

Saleh, M. H., Rashedi, I. and Keating, A., 2017. Immunomodulatory properties of Coriolus versicolor: The role of polysaccharopeptide. *Frontiers in Immunology, 8*, p. 1087.

Brain gym
Stein, M., Federspiel, A., Koenig, T., Wirth, M., Strik, W., Wiest, R., Brandeis, D. and Dierks, T., 2012. Structural plasticity in the language system related to increased second language proficiency. *Cortex, 48*(4), pp. 458–65.

Meditation matters
Xiong, G. L. and Doraiswamy, P. M., 2009. Does meditation enhance cognition and brain plasticity? *Annals of the New York Academy of Sciences, 1172*(1), pp. 63–9.

Brain-boosting moves
Gajjar, A., 19 Jun. 2017. Dementia – and the benefits of dance. Retrieved from https://dramygajjar.com/dementia-and-the-benefits-of-dance/#:~:text=Although%20cognitive%20activity%20reduced%20dementia,a%20staggering%2076%20per%20cent (accessed 29 Sep. 2023).

University of California, 7 Jan. 2022. Exercise alters brain chemistry to protect aging synapses. ScienceDaily. Retrieved from https://www.science-daily.com/releases/2022/01/220107100955.htm (accessed 29 Sep. 2023).

Chapter 9: Movement Matters

Afonso, J., Clemente, F. M., Nakamura, F. Y., Morouço, P., Sarmento, H., Inman, R. A. and Ramirez-Campillo, R., 2021. The effectiveness of post-exercise stretching in short-term and delayed recovery of strength, range of motion and delayed onset muscle soreness: A systematic review and meta-analysis of randomized controlled trials. *Frontiers in Physiology*, p. 553.

Ambrosio, F., Kadi, F., Lexell, J., Fitzgerald, G. K., Boninger, M. L. and Huard, J., 2009. The effect of muscle loading on skeletal muscle regenerative potential: An update of current research findings relating to aging and neuromuscular pathology. *American Journal of Physical Medicine and Rehabilitation, 88*(2), pp. 145–55.

De Brito, L. B. B., Ricardo, D. R., de Araújo, D. S. M. S., Ramos, P. S., Myers, J. and de Araújo, C. G. S., 2014. Ability to sit and rise from the floor as a predictor of all-cause mortality. *European Journal of Preventive Cardiology, 21*(7), pp. 892–8.

Eyre, H. A., Acevedo, B., Yang, H., Siddarth, P., Van Dyk, K., Ercoli, L., Leaver, A. M., Cyr, N. S., Narr, K., Baune, B. T. and Khalsa, D. S., 2016. Changes in neural connectivity and memory following a yoga intervention for older adults: A pilot study. *Journal of Alzheimer's Disease, 52*(2), pp. 673–84.

Frontiers, 23 May 2018. Leg exercise is critical to brain and nervous system health. ScienceDaily. Retrieved from https://www.sciencedaily.com/releases/2018/05/180523080214.htm (accessed 29 Sep. 2023).

Harvard Health Publishing, 1 May 2019. More push-ups may mean less risk of heart problems. Harvard Medical School. Retrieved from https://www.health.harvard.edu/staying-healthy/more-push-ups-may-mean-less-risk-of-heart-problems (accessed 29 Sep. 2023).

Hawke, T. J., 2005. Muscle stem cells and exercise training. *Exercise and Sport Sciences Reviews, 33*(2), pp. 63–8.

He, C., Sumpter, Jr, R. and Levine, B., 2012. Exercise induces autophagy in peripheral tissues and in the brain. *Autophagy, 8*(10), pp. 1548–51.

Kuramoto, K., Liang, H., Hong, J. H. and He, C., 2023. Exercise-activated hepatic autophagy via the FN1-α5β1 integrin pathway drives metabolic benefits of exercise. *Cell Metabolism*, *35*(4), pp. 620–32.

Mitchell, J. J., Blodgett, J. M., Chastin, S. F., Jefferis, B. J., Wannamethee, S. G. and Hamer, M., 2023. Exploring the associations of daily movement behaviours and mid-life cognition: A compositional analysis of the 1970 British Cohort Study. *Journal of Epidemiology and Community Health*, *77*(3), pp. 189–95.

Roberts, H. C., Denison, H. J., Martin, H. J., Patel, H. P., Syddall, H., Cooper, C. and Sayer, A. A., 2011. A review of the measurement of grip strength in clinical and epidemiological studies: Towards a standardised approach. *Age and Ageing*, *40*(4), pp. 423–9.

Wu, M. T., Tang, P. F., Goh, J. O., Chou, T. L., Chang, Y. K., Hsu, Y. C., Chen, Y. J., Chen, N. C., Tseng, W. Y. I., Gau, S. S. F. and Chiu, M. J., 2018. Task-switching performance improvements after Tai Chi Chuan training are associated with greater prefrontal activation in older adults. *Frontiers in Aging Neuroscience*, *10*, p. 280.

Supplements for strength

Buford, T. W., Kreider, R. B., Stout, J. R., Greenwood, M., Campbell, B., Spano, M., Ziegenfuss, T., Lopez, H., Landis, J. and Antonio, J., 2007. International Society of Sports Nutrition position stand: Creatine supplementation and exercise. *Journal of the International Society of Sports Nutrition*, *4*(1), pp. 1–8.

McMorris, T., Mielcarz, G., Harris, R. C., Swain, J. P. and Howard, A., 2007. Creatine supplementation and cognitive performance in elderly individuals. *Aging, Neuropsychology, and Cognition*, *14*(5), pp. 517–28.

Chapter 10: Ways to Rest and Recharge

The importance of sleep

Mashaqi, S. and Gozal, D., 2020. Circadian misalignment and the gut micro-biome. A bidirectional relationship triggering inflammation and metabolic disorders – a literature review. *Sleep Medicine*, *72*, pp. 93–108.

Smith, R. P., Easson, C., Lyle, S. M., Kapoor, R., Donnelly, C. P., Davidson, E. J., Parikh, E., Lopez, J. V. and Tartar, J. L., 2019. Gut microbiome diversity is associated with sleep physiology in humans. *PLoS One, 14*(10), p. e0222394.

Zhou, Q., Zhang, Y., Wang, X., Yang, R., Zhu, X., Zhang, Y., Chen, C., Yuan, H., Yang, Z. and Sun, L., 2020. Gut bacteria Akkermansia is associated with reduced risk of obesity: Evidence from the American Gut Project. *Nutrition and Metabolism, 17*(1), pp. 1–9.

Sleep well
Meredith, S., 27 Sep. 2022. Massive decline in sleep quality in the past year. Medscape UK. Retrieved from https://www.medscape.co.uk/viewarticle/ massive-decline-sleep-quality-across-uk-2022a10023h9 (accessed 29 Sep. 2023).

Sleep problems solved
O'Callaghan, F., Muurlink, O. and Reid, N., 2018. Effects of caffeine on sleep quality and daytime functioning. *Risk Management and Healthcare Policy,* pp. 263–71.

Magnesium
Djokic, G., Vojvodić, P., Korcok, D., Agic, A., Rankovic, A., Djordjevic, V., Vojvodic, A., Vlaskovic-Jovicevic, T., Peric-Hajzler, Z., Matovic, D. and Vojvodic, J., 2019. The effects of magnesium–Melatonin-vit B complex supplementation in treatment of insomnia. *Open Access Macedonian Journal of Medical Sciences, 7*(18), p. 3101.

Mah, J. and Pitre, T., 2021. Oral magnesium supplementation for insomnia in older adults: A systematic review and meta-analysis. *BMC Complementary Medicine and Therapies, 21*(1), pp. 1–11.

Yıldırım, E. and Apaydın, H., 2021. Zinc and magnesium levels of pregnant women with restless leg syndrome and their relationship with anxiety: A case-control study. *Biological Trace Element Research, 199*(5), pp. 1674–85.

L-theanine
Lyon, M. R., Kapoor, M. P. and Juneja, L. R., 2011. The effects of L-theanine (Suntheanine®) on objective sleep quality in boys with attention deficit hyperactivity disorder (ADHD): A randomized, double-blind, placebo-controlled clinical trial. *Alternative Medicine Review, 16*(4), p. 348.

Williams, J., Kellett, J., Roach, P. D., McKune, A., Mellor, D., Thomas, J. and Naumovski, N., 2016. L-theanine as a functional food additive: Its role in disease prevention and health promotion. *Beverages*, 2(2), p. 13.

Montmorency cherry
Losso, J. N., Finley, J. W., Karki, N., Liu, A. G., Prudente, A., Tipton, R., Yu, Y. and Greenway, F. L., 2018. Pilot study of the tart cherry juice for the treatment of insomnia and investigation of mechanisms. *American Journal of Therapeutics*, 25(2), pp. e194-201.

Passiflora
Kim, M., Lim, H. S., Lee, H. H. and Kim, T. H., 2017. Role identification of Passiflora Incarnata Linnaeus: A mini review. *Journal of Menopausal Medicine*, 23(3), pp. 156–9.

Lavender
Koulivand, P. H., Khaleghi Ghadiri, M. and Gorji, A., 2013. Lavender and the nervous system. *Evidence-Based Complementary and Alternative Medicine*.

Lillehei, A. S., Halcón, L. L., Savik, K. and Reis, R., 2015. Effect of inhaled lavender and sleep hygiene on self-reported sleep issues: A randomized controlled trial. *Journal of Alternative and Complementary Medicine*, 21(7), pp. 430–8.

Chamomile
Adib-Hajbaghery, M. and Mousavi, S. N., 2017. The effects of chamomile extract on sleep quality among elderly people: A clinical trial. *Complementary Therapies in Medicine*, 35, pp. 109–14.

Valerian
Shinjyo, N., Waddell, G. and Green, J., 2020. Valerian root in treating sleep problems and associated disorders – A systematic review and meta-analysis. *Journal of Evidence-Based Integrative Medicine*, 25, p. 2515690X20967323.

CBD

Boehnke, K. F., Gagnier, J. J., Matallana, L. and Williams, D. A., 2021. Cannabidiol use for fibromyalgia: Prevalence of use and perceptions of effectiveness in a large online survey. *Journal of Pain*, 22(5), pp. 556–66.

Ranum, R. M., Whipple, M. O., Croghan, I., Bauer, B., Toussaint, L. L. and Vincent, A., 2023. Use of cannabidiol in the management of insomnia: A systematic review. *Cannabis and Cannabinoid Research*, 8(2), pp. 213–29.

Shannon, S., Lewis, N., Lee, H. and Hughes, S., 2019. Cannabidiol in anxiety and sleep: A large case series. *Permanente Journal*, 23.

Silvestro, S., Mammana, S., Cavalli, E., Bramanti, P. and Mazzon, E., 2019. Use of cannabidiol in the treatment of epilepsy: Efficacy and security in clinical trials. *Molecules*, 24(8), p. 1459.

Chapter 11: The Power of Connection

Koenig, H. G., 2012. Religion, spirituality, and health: The research and clinical implications. *International Scholarly Research Notices*, 2012.

National Academies of Sciences, Engineering, and Medicine, 2020. *Social Isolation and Loneliness In Older Adults: Opportunities for the Health Care System*. National Academies Press.

Sex talk

Brody, S., 2010. The relative health benefits of different sexual activities. *The Journal of Sexual Medicine*, 7(4_Part_1), pp. 1336–61.

Charnetski, C. J. and Brennan, F. X., 2004. Sexual frequency and salivary immunoglobulin A (IgA). *Psychological Reports*, 94(3), pp. 839–44.

Gratitude goals

UC Davis Health Medical Center, 25 Nov. 2015. Gratitude is good medicine. Retrieved from https://health.ucdavis.edu/medicalcenter/features/2015-2016/11/20151125_gratitude.html#:~:text="It%20can%20lower%20blood%20pressure,Practicing%20gratitude%20also%20affects%20behavior (accessed 29 Sep. 2023).

Chapter 12: Beauty Bio-Hacks

Resveratrol

Granzotto, A. and Zatta, P., 2014. Resveratrol and Alzheimer's disease: Message in a bottle on red wine and cognition. *Frontiers in Aging Neuroscience*, 6, p. 95.

Kuršvietienė, L., Stanevičienė, I., Mongirdienė, A. and Bernatonienė, J., 2016. Multiplicity of effects and health benefits of resveratrol. *Medicina*, 52(3), pp. 148–55.

Liu, Y., Ma, W., Zhang, P., He, S. and Huang, D., 2015. Effect of resveratrol on blood pressure: A meta-analysis of randomized controlled trials. *Clinical Nutrition*, 34(1), pp. 27–34.

Moussa, C., Hebron, M., Huang, X., Ahn, J., Rissman, R. A., Aisen, P. S. and Turner, R. S., 2017. Resveratrol regulates neuro-inflammation and induces adaptive immunity in Alzheimer's disease. *Journal of Neuroinflammation*, 14, pp. 1–10.

Vallianou, N. G., Evangelopoulos, A. and Kazazis, C., 2013. Resveratrol and diabetes. *Review of Diabetic Studies: RDS*, 10(4), p. 236.

NAD+

Hubbard, B. P., Gomes, A. P., Dai, H., Li, J., Case, A. W., Considine, T., Riera, T. V., Lee, J. E., E, S. Y., Lamming, D. W. and Pentelute, B. L., 2013. Evidence for a common mechanism of SIRT1 regulation by allosteric activators. *Science*, 339(6124), pp. 1216–19.

McReynolds, M. R., Chellappa, K. and Baur, J. A., 2020. Age-related NAD+ decline. *Experimental Gerontology*, 134, p. 110888.

Miranda, D. R., 21 Jun. 2022. Australian scientists find exercise boosts NAD+ in young but not older adults. NAD+ Aging Science. Retrieved from https://www.nad.com/news/exercise-boosts-nad# (accessed 29 Sep. 2023).

Lamb, D. A., Moore, J. H., Mesquita, P. H. C., Smith, M. A., Vann, C. G., Osburn, S. C., Fox, C. D., Lopez, H. L., Ziegenfuss, T. N., Huggins, K. W. and Goodlett, M. D., 2020. Resistance training increases muscle NAD+ and NADH concentrations as well as NAMPT protein levels and global sirtuin activity in middle-aged, overweight, untrained individuals. *Aging (Albany NY)*, 12(10), p. 9447.

Quercetin

Cui, Z., Zhao, X., Amevor, F. K., Du, X., Wang, Y., Li, D., Shu, G., Tian, Y. and Zhao, X., 2022. Therapeutic application of quercetin in aging-related diseases: SIRT1 as a potential mechanism. *Frontiers in Immunology*, *13*, p. 943321.

Making sense of methylation

Christensen, B. C., Kelsey, K. T., Zheng, S., Houseman, E. A., Marsit, C.J., Wrensch, M. R., Wiemels, J. L., Nelson, H. H., Karagas, M. R., Kushi, L. H., Kwan, M. L. and Wiencke, J. K., 2010. Breast cancer DNA methylation profiles are associated with tumor size and alcohol and folate intake. *PLOS Genetics*, *6*(7), p. e1001043.

ElGendy, K., Malcomson, F. C., Lara, J. G., Bradburn, D. M. and Mathers, J. C., 2018. Effects of dietary interventions on DNA methylation in adult humans: Systematic review and meta-analysis. *British Journal of Nutrition*, *120*(9), pp. 961–76.

Phillips, T., 2008. The role of methylation in gene expression. *Nature Education*, *1*(1), p. 116.

Pro-ageing skincare

Pillaiyar, T., Manickam, M. and Namasivayam, V., 2017. Skin whitening agents: Medicinal chemistry perspective of tyrosinase inhibitors. *Journal of Enzyme Inhibition and Medicinal Chemistry*, *32*(1), pp. 403–25.

Acknowledgements

The concept of *A Better Second Half* came out of conversations I was having with my publishing team at Liz Earle Wellbeing, as I wanted to move the conversation on from simply talking about 'wellbeing' and be more specific. I wanted us to be able to offer more help for midlife women, too often let down by unresolved health issues, unhelped by declining hormones, circumstance and life changes. Having been through times of change myself – and found ways to renew and thrive – I said I was at last having a 'better second half' and wanted the same for all. At that moment, the concept of this book was born.

I am supremely grateful to my literary agent, the powerhouse that is Carly Cook, for not only running with my idea, but bringing it to the incredible team at Yellow Kite books. It's been a privilege to work with such a talented group of professionals, from Carolyn Thorne, my inspirational publisher, to Julia Kellaway, my genius editor. I later discovered that Julia had edited one of my first books, *New Vital Oils*, so it seemed just right that we were now working together on this – much more advanced work – so many years later. I am grateful for the additional research undertaken by Freya Millis, always undaunted when I threw a new topic her way with a request to investigate. Between us, we discerned much of the woo-woo noise from the strategies that bear stricter scrutiny, however strange they might sound – such as cold showers and grounding!

I'm also indebted to my top team at Liz Earle Wellbeing, whose tireless enthusiasm and support for all we do in the wellness space never ceases to inspire and encourage me. In particular, Polly Beard, Sara Munds, Ellie Smith, Amy Moore, Rachel Andrews, Betty Beard, and Leni Syndica-Drummond (who took the book jacket photo of me and many more featured here).

Also, to the many specialists and experts who have so kindly guided me through the complex maze of medical matters and beyond, helping to ensure the information in this book is as accurate and reliable as it can be. These include Tom Baxter, Lucy Beresford, Emma Beswick, Prof Avrum Bluming, Nichola Conlon, James Earl, Dr Jason Fung, Michael Garry, Zoe Harcombe, Ed van Harmelen, Jillian Lavender, Dr Aseem Malholtra, Dr Louise Newson and Megan Ramos.

To my five children, for their unstinting support and generosity in giving me the time to follow my purpose in writing this book, inevitably taking time away from them. I hope they find it a worthy legacy and blueprint for their own lives in the future. To CJ, the man who has supported me through so much of my later writing and been an inspiration for my own personal second half – making it not only better, but complete.

Last, but not least, I would like to thank the incredible Liz Earle Wellbeing community who join me daily across all forms of social media, generously sharing ideas, exchanging views and generally supporting the sisterhood. Together we are stronger and together we can be the change to ensure a 'better second half' for us all.

Index

D
daily routine 27–39
dairy foods 145–9
Davis, Dr William 209
deep vein thrombosis (DVT) 84
dehydration 188, 189
dementia 15, 41, 106, 226–7, 228–9, 271
dental floss 30–1
dermablading 299, 300
diabetes 94, 102, 130, 136, 170, 174–5, 184, 210
diet 15, 109–68
   80:20 rule 171
   carbohydrates 130–4, 174
   chocolate 160–3
   eggs 149–51
   fats 110–30
   fish 152–6, 159
   fruit and vegetables 156–7, 158, 166
   junk food 144
   kitchen cupboard staples 166–7
   low-carb diet 174
   meat 158, 159
   and menopause 99–105
   milk and dairy foods 145–9
   nutrigenomics 49–52
   and oestrogen 212
   protein 134–43
   and sleep 262
   snacks 165–6
   sugars 177–81
   timing 135
dieting 170–1, 174
digestion: gut health and 211
   and sleep 258
divorce 274–5, 281
DNA: methylation 291–2
   nutrigenomics 49–52
   telomere length 47, 48, 61, 193
docosahexaenoic acid (DHA) 105, 125, 140,
   155, 226–7
doctors 43–4
dong quai 87, 98
dopamine 49–50, 196, 208, 223
drinks 187–207
   alcohol 202–6
   coffee 50, 189, 191–5
   diet drinks 179
   electrolytes 187, 188–91
   tea 183, 189, 196–202, 264–5
   time-restricted eating 176
   water 187–8
drippings 116, 122
drugs: women's response to 39–40

see also hormone replacement therapy
   (HRT)

E
early rising 261
eating disorders 173
eggs 149–51
eicosapentaenoic acid (EPA) 105, 125, 139–40,
   155, 227
electrolytes 32, 187, 188–91
endometriosis 40, 41, 85
endorphins 106, 161
energy, mitochondria 62
enzymes 62
epicatechin 160–1
epigenetics 14, 291
essential fatty acids 99, 116
estrogen see oestrogen
ethanol 202
eucalyptus fibre bedding 267
exercise 16, 241–55
   and autophagy 59
   and blood pressure 131
   and brain 238–9
   daily routine 37–8
   and glutathione 69–70
   guidelines 242
   running 243–5
   and sleep 260
   and supplements 253–5
   ten-minute guide 54, 245–9
   weightlifting 251–3
exosomes 299

F
face: injectable face treatments 298–9
   LED-light and laser facials 297–8
   non-surgical face lifts 300–1
fasting 203
   and autophagy 58–9, 60
   intermittent 54, 221
   non-surgical face lifts 299–300
   time-restricted eating 174–6, 221, 225
fat: abdominal 84, 134–5, 170
   autophagy 58
   fat metabolism 53, 58
fats, dietary 99–100, 110–30, 240
fennel seed tea 199
fermented foods 209, 215–21
fibre 132, 134, 184–5, 209, 214
fillers, injectable 298–9
fish 152–6, 159
fish oils 105, 125, 226–8

Picture Acknowledgements

The author and publisher would like to thank the following copyright holders for permission to reproduce images in this book:

1. This Morning/ITV Studios
2. BBC Books
3. BBC Books
4. Author's collection
5. Iain Philpott
6. News International
7. Author's collection
8. Author's collection
9. Author's collection
10. Author's collection
11. Patrick Drummond
12. Georgia Glynn Smith
13. Leni's Lens
14. Leni's Lens
15. Leni's Lens
16. Kit Drummond
17. Leni's Lens

18. Leni's Lens
19. Leni's Lens
20. Leni's Lens
21. Leni's Lens
22. Leni's Lens
23. Red Rabbit Photography
24. Leni's Lens

About the Author

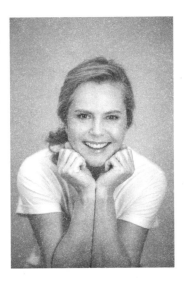

Liz Earle MBE is one of the UK's most trusted authorities on wellbeing. An award-winning author of over 30 books on nutrition, diet, beauty, gut health, hormone health and natural wellness, she co-founded the highly successful Liz Earle Beauty Co. in 1995 before moving back to writing and broadcasting. She hosts the popular *Liz Earle Wellbeing Show* and is a regular commentator on TV and radio.

An expert in mid-life living and longevity, her straightforward, balanced and well-researched approach has earned her a place as a trusted visionary in the world of wellbeing. With a passion for demystifying science and sharing tried-and-tested wellness wisdom, Liz's measured voice of reason has a deservedly large and loyal following in print, on digital and online. Travelling the globe both for research and for the humanitarian charity she founded in 2010, LiveTwice, Liz is also an ambassador and advocate for many environmental and healthcare charities including Ace Africa, Compassion in World Farming, International Health partners, Love British Food, The Menopause Charity, The Royal Countryside Fund, The Royal Osteoporosis Society, The Sustainable Food Trust and Tearfund.

lizearlewellbeing.com